POCKET
GUIDE TO  IBD

SECOND EDITION

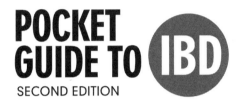

POCKET GUIDE TO IBD
SECOND EDITION

Edited by

Marla Dubinsky, MD
Associate Professor of Pediatrics
Director of the Pediatric IBD Center
Cedars-Sinai Medical Center
Los Angeles, California

Sonia Friedman, MD, FACG
Assistant Professor of Medicine
Harvard Medical School
Brigham and Women's Hospital
Boston, Massachusetts

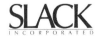

SLACK
INCORPORATED

www.slackbooks.com

ISBN: 978-1-55642-991-0

Copyright © 2011 by SLACK Incorporated

The previous edition of *Pocket Guide to IBD* was published in 2005 by Cambridge University Press.

Published by: SLACK Incorporated
                  6900 Grove Road
                  Thorofare, NJ 08086 USA
                  Telephone: 856-848-1000
                  Fax: 856-848-6091
                  www.slackbooks.com

Contact SLACK Incorporated for more information about other books in this field or about the availability of our books from distributors outside the United States.

Library of Congress Cataloging-in-Publication Data

Pocket guide to IBD / [edited by] Marla Dubinsky, MD, Associate Professor of Pediatrics, Director of the Pediatric IBD Center, Cedars-Sinai Medical Center, Los Angeles, CA, Sonia Friedman, MD, FACP, Assistant Professor of Medicine, Harvard Medical School, Brigham and Women's Hospital, Boston, MA. -- Second Edition.
   p. ; cm.
   IBD
   Inflammatory bowel disease
   Includes bibliographical references and index.
   ISBN 978-1-55642-991-0 (alk. paper)
   1. Inflammatory bowel diseases--Handbooks, manuals, etc. I. Dubinsky, Marla C., 1967- editor. II. Friedman, Sonia, 1966- editor. III. Pocket guide to inflammatory bowel disease. Revision of (work): IV. Title: IBD. V. Title: Inflammatory bowel disease.
   [DNLM: 1. Inflammatory Bowel Diseases--Handbooks. WI 39]
   RC862.I53P63 2011
   616.3'44--dc22
                              2010052025

Printed in the United States of America.

Last digit is print number: 10 9   8   7   6   5   4   3   2   1

Dedication

We would like to dedicate this book to our IBD patients and their families.

Contents

Acknowledgments

We would like to thank all the contributors who took time out of their very busy schedules to help bring this book to life. Their practical approach to the management of IBD has been transcribed in the pages of the *Pocket Guide* and helps make this book a great guide for the reader. We would like to also acknowledge all of our teachers and mentors who have influenced us along the way and continue to help guide our careers.

About the Editors

Marla Dubinsky, MD received a medical degree from Queen's University in Canada and completed her clinical pediatric gastroenterology training at Sainte-Justine Hospital, University of Montreal in Quebec, Canada. Currently, Dr. Dubinsky is Director of the Pediatric Inflammatory Bowel Disease Center at Cedars-Sinai Medical Center in Los Angeles, CA. In addition, Dr. Dubinsky is Associate Professor of Pediatrics at the University of California, Los Angeles, David Geffen School of Medicine.

Board certified in pediatrics and pediatric gastroenterology, Dr. Dubinsky holds positions of prominence with several advisory bodies, including Chair of the Western Regional Pediatric IBD Research Alliance. She is a member of several professional societies, including the American Gastroenterology Association, the American College of Gastroenterology, and the American Academy of Pediatrics. Among her many awards, Dr. Dubinsky was a Crohn's and Colitis Foundation of America Medical Honoree in 2004 and recently received the Lenny and Corinne Sands Clinical Investigator Award.

Dr. Dubinsky's main research interests are health outcomes and the epidemiology and genetic influences of inflammatory bowel disease (IBD) in children. Her objective is to study the influence of genetics and immune responses on the variability in clinical presentations of early-onset IBD. Additional interests include the study of pharmacogenetics to evaluate how heredity influences drug responses and optimizing and individualizing the management of IBD. Dr. Dubinsky's work has been published in numerous peer-reviewed journals, including *Gastroenterology, The Journal of Pediatric Gastroenterology and Nutrition, Inflammatory Bowel Diseases,* and *The American Journal of Gastroenterology*. In addition, she has authored book chapters for *Trends in Inflammatory Bowel Disease Therapy and Inflammatory Bowel Disease: Diagnosis and Therapeutics*. Dr. Dubinsky has lectured widely both nationally and internationally.

Sonia Friedman, MD, FACG completed her undergraduate degree in biology at Stanford University in California and her medical degree at Yale University School of Medicine. She completed her medical internship and residency at University of Pennsylvania and her gastroenterology fellowship at Mount Sinai Medical Center in New York City. She specialized in IBD during her fellowship and now has a large IBD practice in the gastroenterology division of Brigham and Women's Hospital. She has been at Brigham and Women's for the past 11 years and is Director of IBD Clinical Research.

Dr. Friedman's research interests include colon cancer in Crohn's disease, patient adherence to surveillance colonoscopy, and IBD and pregnancy.

She is a section editor for *Inflammatory Bowel Diseases* and a reviewer for *Gastroenterology, Clinical Gastroenterology and Hepatology,* and *The American Journal of Gastroenterology*. Dr. Friedman has published mainly on colonoscopic surveillance in Crohn's colitis and IBD in pregnancy and also enjoys lecturing on these subjects.

Dr. Friedman is chair of the Crohn's and Colitis Foundation, New England Chapter Medical Advisory Committee. She has been elected as "Best Up and Coming Gastroenterologist in Boston" in 2004 and also listed as "Best of Boston" in *Boston* magazine in 2007. Both honors are based on peer review.

Contributing Authors

Maria T. Abreu, MD (Chapter 2)
Professor of Medicine
Chief, Division of Gastroenterology
University of Miami, Miller School of Medicine
Miami, Florida

David G. Binion, MD (Appendix B)
Co-Director, Inflammatory Bowel Disease Center
Director, Translational Inflammatory Bowel Disease Research
Visiting Professor of Medicine
Division of Gastroenterology, Hepatology, and Nutrition
University of Pittsburgh, School of Medicine
Pittsburgh, Pennsylvania

Russell D. Cohen, MD, FACG, AGAF (Chapter 1)
Associate Professor of Medicine
Pritzker School of Medicine
Co-Director, Inflammatory Bowel Disease Center
The University of Chicago Medical Center
Chicago, Illinois

Judy F. Collins, MD (Chapter 13)
Associate Professor of Medicine
Oregon Health and Sciences University
Section Chief, Gastroenterology, Portland VA Medical Center
Portland, Oregon

Erin Feldman, RD, CSP (Chapter 20)
Clinical Dietitian
Pediatric IBD Center
Cedars Sinai Medical Center
Los Angeles, California

Sandra M. El-Hachem, MD (Appendix B)
Clinical Assistant Professor of Medicine
Division of Gastroenterology, Hepatology and Nutrition
University of Pittsburgh Medical Center
Pittsburgh, Pennsylvania

Matthew J. Hamilton, MD (Chapter 18)
Instructor of Medicine
Harvard Medical School
Division of Gastroenterology
Brigham and Women's Hospital
Boston, Massachusetts

Debra J. Helper, MD (Chapter 8)
Associate Professor of Clinical Medicine
Medical Director, Inflammatory Bowel Disease Center
Division of Gastroenterology/Hepatology
Indiana University School of Medicine
Indianapolis, Indiana

Sarah N. Horst, MD (Chapter 10)
Fellow, Gastroenterology
Digestive Disease Center
Vanderbilt University Medical Center
Nashville, Tennessee

Kim L. Isaacs, MD, PhD (Chapters 7 and 11)
Professor of Medicine
Division of Gastroenterology and Hepatology
University of North Carolina at Chapel Hill
Chapel Hill, North Carolina

Sunanda V. Kane, MD, MSPH, FACG, FACP, AGAF
(Chapters 3, 9, 22, and Appendix A)
Professor of Medicine
Division of Gastroenterology and Hepatology
Mayo Clinic College of Medicine
Rochester, Minnesota

Joshua Korzenik, MD (Chapter 12)
Inflammatory Bowel Disease Center
Gastrointestinal Unit
Massachusetts General Hospital
Boston, Massachusetts

Edward V. Loftus Jr, MD (Chapter 21)
Professor of Medicine
Chair, Inflammatory Bowel Disease Interest Group
Division of Gastroenterology and Hepatology
Mayo Clinic
Rochester, Minnesota

Uma Mahadevan, MD (Chapter 17)
Associate Professor of Medicine
Center for Colitis and Crohn's Disease
University of California, San Francisco
San Francisco, California

Nimisha K. Parekh, MD (Chapter 15)
Director, Inflammatory Bowel Disease Program
H. H. Chao Comprehensive Digestive Disease Center
Assistant Clinical Professor of Medicine
Department of Medicine
University of California, Irvine
Irvine, California

David T. Rubin, MD, FACG, AGAF (Chapter 19)
Associate Professor of Medicine
Co-Director, Inflammatory Bowel Disease Center
University of Chicago Medical Center
Chicago, Illinois

Ellen J. Scherl, MD (Chapter 4)
Director, Inflammatory Bowel Disease Center
Weill Cornell Medical College
New York, New York

David A. Schwartz, MD (Chapter 10)
Director, Inflammatory Bowel Disease Center
Associate Professor of Medicine
Vanderbilt University Medical Center
Nashville, Tennessee

Bo Shen, MD (Chapter 14)
Assistant Professor of Medicine
Section Head
Department of Gastroenterology and Hepatology
Cleveland Clinic
Cleveland, Ohio

Preface

There are many excellent books available that address the pathophysiology, epidemiology, and detailed treatment approaches to IBD. Sometimes, however, we want a user-friendly resource to address common clinical scenarios that we encounter every day in our clinics and on the wards. The *Pocket Guide to IBD* was designed specifically for busy clinicians and trainees who want easy access to the key diagnostic and treatment considerations when faced with an IBD patient. This book summarizes the key clinical symptoms and scenarios as well as differential diagnoses a clinician may encounter when managing an IBD patient and provides practical decision-making information. To address the needs of special IBD populations such as children, pregnant women, and the elderly, the chapters highlight the key elements to managing these patients. The short chapter format and the accompanying tables and figures provide clinicians with a quick reference guide for common topics in IBD and also draw attention to important areas such as complementary and alternative medicine, management of stomas, and colon cancer screening.

Introduction

It can be difficult for the practicing gastroenterologist, physician assistant, or nurse practitioner to keep up with the variety and complexities of today's IBD treatments. Thankfully, there are multiple ongoing clinical trials in IBD, and treatment algorithms are frequently being updated. Given the success of the new biologic medications, it is important for practitioners to be comfortable with both new and old IBD therapies and familiar with their risks, side effects, and complications. The number of IBD patients we see is continually increasing, and our office practices are getting busier with less time for us to look up the latest recommendations. The *Pocket Guide to IBD* is a great resource for practitioners who need quick and accurate answers to all important questions relevant to IBD. Each concise chapter contains bullet points and clear tables and figures that quickly and comprehensively illustrate each subject. We think that this essential resource will fill any gaps in IBD knowledge, great or small, and help improve the everyday care of patients with Crohn's disease and ulcerative colitis.

Foreword

The Roman poet Horace (Quintus Horatius Flaccus, 65 B.C.–8 B.C.) said, "Whatever advice you give, be short." Clearly, the editors and contributors of this second edition of the *Pocket Guide to IBD* have adhered to Horace's dictum. Eschewing detailed expositions of pathophysiology and florid descriptions of obscure literature, this little book asks the question, "What does one really need to know about IBD?"—and then answers it. Contained within, the reader will find the practical knowledge that every clinician requires when caring for the patient with Crohn's disease or ulcerative colitis. Organized by symptom, therapy, and special populations or considerations, the book provides a matrix of information that permits a comprehensive approach while remaining brief. In many cases, charts and flow diagrams beautifully illuminate the text, further enhancing the usefulness of this work. In short, few books on IBD have covered so much material, so well, in so few words.

Bruce Sands, MD, MS
Chief, Henry D. Janowitz Division of Gastroenterology
Mount Sinai Medical Center
New York, NY

SECTION I

BASIC OVERVIEWS

Introduction to
Ulcerative Colitis

Russell D. Cohen, MD, FACG, AGAF

Ulcerative colitis (UC) is one of the 2 major groups of chronic idiopathic inflammatory bowel disease. UC is a worldwide disorder that primarily affects young adults between the ages of 20 and 40 years, but the disease may present at any age. There appears to be a genetic susceptibility, which is only partly understood. Certain racial and ethnic groups tend to more prone to UC than other groups. The familial incidence of UC has been recognized for many years, but specific genes have yet to be identified. The cause remains unknown, but environmental, immunologic, and psychological factors are thought to be contributors to the etiology and pathogenesis of UC. For example, appendectomy in childhood protects against the future development of UC. Another intriguing factor is that UC is primarily a disease of nonsmokers; smokers are protected against UC . . . until they quit.

Dubinsky M, Friedman S.
Pocket Guide to IBD, Second Edition (pp 3-8).
© 2011 SLACK Incorporated

Clinical Features

The major symptoms of UC include diarrhea, rectal bleeding, and abdominal pain. Disease of moderate or severe activity may be associated with systemic symptoms such as anorexia, nausea, vomiting, fever, and fatigue. Extraintestinal manifestations include arthritis, skin changes such as pyoderma gangrenosum and erythema nodosum, eye changes, and evidence of liver disease. Some of these extracolonic findings are related to the activity of the colitis and resolve when the colonic inflammation is controlled. Endoscopically, inflammation begins in the rectum and extends proximally in a continuous and circumferential fashion, without "skip areas." Approximately one-third of patients will have colitis extending proximally beyond the splenic flexure (or beyond 60 cm, as measured from the anal verge), one-third will have disease extending up to but not beyond the splenic flexure, and another one-third will have disease limited to just the rectum (Table 1-1).

Complications

Patients with active colitis can suffer from anemia, dehydration, and electrolyte disorders. Chronically ill patients may be prone to venous thrombosis, anemia, weight loss, and a chronically scarred colon that is refractory to medical therapies and antidiarrheals. Severe complications may include massive hemorrhage, perforation, and toxic megacolon. Patients with chronic colitis are at a higher risk for colorectal cancer and require periodic surveillance colonoscopies.

Therapy

The initial treatment for UC is usually medical (Table 1-2); surgery is reserved for patients with intractable disease,

Table 1-1. Classification of Ulcerative Colitis

Disease Location	Upper Extent of Inflammation[†]	Colon Cancer Risk[††]	First-Line Therapies
Proctitis	Rectum (10 cm)	Not increased	Suppository/foam
Left-sided colitis*	Splenic flexure (60 cm)	Slight increase	Enema ± oral
Extensive colitis**	Beyond splenic flexure (>60 cm)	Greater increase	Oral ± enema

*Disease extending to the proximal sigmoid is subclassified as "proctosigmoiditis."
**Disease extending to the cecum is subclassified as "pancolitis."
[†]As measured from the anal verge.
[††]As compared to age-matched controls not otherwise classified as high-risk.

Table 1-2. Medical Therapies Used in Ulcerative Colitis

Disease Severity	Choice of Therapies
Mild	Aminosalicylates: oral ± topical Corticosteroids: topical*

Moderate
  Acute
  Steroid-dependent
  Steroid-refractory[†]
	Corticosteroids: oral ± topical*
	Aminosalicylates: oral ± topical
	Azathioprine/6-mercaptopurine
	Infliximab/other anti-tumor necrosis factor agents

Severe
  Acute
  Intravenous steroid-refractory[†]
	Intravenous corticosteroids*
	Cyclosporine/tacrolimus/infliximab

*Corticosteroid use appropriate only for short-term therapy.
[†]Surgical consultation recommended/required.

complications of corticosteroid dependence, or colorectal dysplasia or cancer. First-line medical therapies include the aminosalicylates (sulfasalazine, mesalamine, balsalazide, and olsalazine). Patients refractory to these agents often are treated initially with systemic corticosteroids; those with corticosteroid-dependent disease are subsequently started on a purine analog (azathioprine or 6-mercaptopurine). Failure of these therapies often heralds the introduction of a therapy targeting tumor necrosis factor (infliximab) or surgery. Cyclosporine or tacrolimus is used for disease that is refractory to high-dose oral or intravenous steroids.

Endoscopic assessment of disease extent and severity is helpful in effective management. Disease limited to the rectum or rectosigmoid may be managed with medicated suppositories, foams, or enemas. More extensive disease requires the addition of oral therapies. Mild to moderately active disease can usually be treated on an outpatient basis. More severe disease may require treatment in the hospital setting, and surgical consultation is recommended.

The principal drugs used in the therapy of UC are the aminosalicylates (sulfasalazine, mesalamine, balsalazide, and olsalazine; this class is referred to as 5-ASA compounds), corticosteroids, and immunosuppressives (azathioprine, 6-mercaptopurine, and cyclosporine). Once the disease is in remission, patients are usually maintained with 5-ASAs or purine metabolites (azathioprine and 6-mercaptopurine).

Approximately 20% to 25% of patients will require colectomy during the course of the disease. Indications for colectomy include severe attacks failing to respond to medical therapy, complications of a severe attack, chronic continuous disease with impaired quality of life, dysplasia, and carcinoma.

Prognosis

Most patients with UC have intermittent attacks of their disease. A few patients will have only a single attack. Approximately 10% to 15% of patients will have a chronic continuous course. Patients with extensive colitis, or pancolitis, are much more likely to have severe attacks than those patients with limited disease, have higher risk for colon cancer, and are more likely to require surgery over their lifetime. The life expectancy of patients with UC is roughly the same as that for the general population.

SUGGESTED READINGS

Farmer RG, Easley KA, Rankin GB. Clinical patterns, natural history, and progression of ulcerative colitis: a long-term follow-up of 1116 patients. *Dig Dis Sci.* 1993;38(6):1137-1346.

Hanauer SB, Sandborn WJ, Kornbluth A, et al. Delayed-release oral mesalamine at 4.8 g/day (800 mg tablet) for the treatment of moderately active ulcerative colitis: the ASCEND II trial. *Am J Gastroenterol.* 2005;100(11):2478-2485.

Hawthorne AB, Logan RF, Hawkey CJ, et al. Randomised controlled trial of azathioprine withdrawal in ulcerative colitis. *BMJ.* 1992;305(6844):20-22.

Kornbluth A, Sachar DB. Ulcerative colitis practice guidelines in adults (update): American College of Gastroenterology, Practice Parameters Committee. *Am J Gastroenterol.* 2004;99(7):1371-1385.

Langholz E, Munkholm P, Davidsen M, Binder V. Colorectal cancer risk and mortality in patients with ulcerative colitis. *Gastroenterology.* 1992;103(5):1444-1451.

Lichtiger S, Present DH, Kornbluth A, et al. Cyclosporine in severe ulcerative colitis refractory to steroid therapy. *N Engl J Med.* 1994;330(26):1841-1845.

Loftus EV Jr. Clinical epidemiology of inflammatory bowel disease: incidence, prevalence, and environmental influences. *Gastroenterology.* 2004;126(6):1504-1517.

Rutgeerts P, Sandborn WJ, Feagan BG, et al. Infliximab for induction and maintenance therapy for ulcerative colitis. *N Engl J Med.* 2005;353(23):2462-2476.

2

Introduction to Crohn's Disease

Maria T. Abreu, MD

Crohn's disease (CD) is a chronic IBD involving the gastrointestinal tract that can manifest in a variety of ways and is characterized by episodes of acute flares of symptoms and periods of remission. CD may be diagnosed at any age but is commonly diagnosed in young adults. It is more common in industrialized nations in northern climates, with the highest prevalence found in northern Europe, the United Kingdom, and North America. The prevalence of CD in the United States ranges from 26 to 199 cases per 100,000 persons. It affects all ethnic groups but is more common in White populations and carries a slightly greater risk in the Jewish population, especially in persons with Jewish European descent. The incidence of CD in African Americans and Latinos also has been rising in recent years. The cause of the disease is not entirely understood, but it is likely the result of an individual's genetic makeup and environmental exposures.

9

Dubinsky M, Friedman S.
Pocket Guide to IBD, Second Edition (pp 9-12).
© 2011 SLACK Incorporated

Clinical Features

CD may involve any portion of the gastrointestinal tract from the mouth to the anus. Most commonly, however, it affects the terminal ileum and some part of the colon. In up to 30% of cases, CD is located only in the colon and may occasionally be confused with ulcerative colitis. The inflammation in CD is typically discontinuous, with areas of normal mucosa in-between areas of inflamed mucosa. The inflammation may involve the full thickness of the bowel wall, which can lead to the development of large and deep ulcerations and fistulas. Many complications can potentially result from the inflammatory process found in CD. Chronic inflammation can lead to stricturing of the bowel lumen, sometimes resulting in bowel obstruction. Abscesses or fistulas, connections between the intestines and another loop of bowel, the bladder, vagina, or skin may also develop.

Symptoms of CD vary depending on the location of disease involvement and the extent and severity of inflammation. In fact, CD is often categorized by disease location and disease behavior. Disease behavior can be described as predominantly inflammatory, fibrostenotic, or penetrating in nature. Patients may experience abdominal pain, diarrhea, fever, weight loss, or fatigue. Some patients develop perianal abscesses or fistulas to the skin surrounding the anus. Patients may also experience extraintestinal manifestations such as arthritis, skin rashes including pyoderma gangrenosum and erythema nodosum, inflammation of the eye, and diseases involving the liver.

Therapy

Treatment of CD depends on disease location and the severity of disease. There are 2 stages of therapy in the treatment of IBD, the induction of remission and the maintenance of remission. Aminosalicylate preparations

(5-ASAs) are sometimes used for the treatment of active disease and the maintenance of remission but are the weakest therapies available. Antibiotics are also used to treat active disease, especially colonic CD. Corticosteroids are sometimes needed on a short-term basis to induce remission. Newer corticosteroids, such as enteric-coated budesonide, have fewer systemic side effects and can be used to treat ileocolonic mild to moderate CD. Many patients require treatment with immunomodulators, such as azathioprine or 6-mercaptopurine. These medications are used as maintenance drugs in patients who have mild to moderate disease or steroid-dependent disease.

The big advance in CD therapy has been biologic drugs. At least for now, these targeted therapies block tumor necrosis factor (TNF)-alpha and are termed *anti-TNFs*. Currently, 3 anti-TNFs are approved for induction and maintenance of remission in CD—infliximab, adalimumab, and certolizumab. Although head-to-head studies have not been performed, all 3 of these agents appear to be similarly effective and have similar side effects. Only infliximab is approved for the treatment of perianal fistulas. Surgery remains an important therapeutic option when medical therapy has failed.

Prognosis

CD is a lifelong disease, but with proper diagnosis and management of the disease and its complications, patients often lead healthy and normal lives. Several recent studies have shown that earlier use of biologics alone or in combination with an immunomodulator can alter the progression of CD.

Suggested Readings

Bayless TM, Hanauer SB, eds. *Advanced Therapy of Inflammatory Bowel Disease*. Hamilton, Ontario: BC Decker Incorporated; 2001.

Kane SV. IBD *Self-Management: The AGA Guide to Crohn's Disease and Ulcerative Colitis*. Bethesda, MD: AGA Press; 2010.

Targan SR, Shanahan F, Karp LC. *Inflammatory Bowel Disease: Translating Basic Science Into Clinical Practice*. Hoboken, NJ: Wiley-Blackwell; 2010.

SECTION II

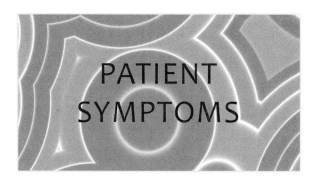

PATIENT
SYMPTOMS

Abdominal Pain

Sunanda V. Kane, MD, MSPH, FACG, FACP, AGAF

Abdominal pain is a common occurrence in patients with IBD. It often can be caused by a flare or a complication of IBD. Non–IBD-related conditions such as acute appendicitis and irritable bowel syndrome can also cause abdominal pain. Sometimes it can be tricky to distinguish between IBD and non–IBD-related etiologies.

I. CONDITIONS TO CONSIDER

- In Crohn's disease
  - Acute obstruction (partial or complete bowel obstruction)
  - Perforation
  - Abscess
  - Active inflammatory disease

- In ulcerative colitis
  - Severe colitis
  - Perforation
  - Toxic megacolon

Dubinsky M, Friedman S.
Pocket Guide to IBD, Second Edition (pp 15-18).
© 2011 SLACK Incorporated

- In either diagnosis
  - Peptic ulcer disease
  - Pancreatitis
  - Gallstones, kidney stones
  - Acute appendicitis
  - Medication-related pain
  - Irritable bowel syndrome
  - Diverticulosis
  - Infection

II. Questions to Ask

Where is the pain?

- The location can help determine the etiology.

What is the character of the pain (eg, crampy, colicky, diffuse, sharp)?

How long has the pain been present?

- Pain present for a few days rules out an acute, emergent situation.

Is the pain related to oral intake?

Is there anything that relieves the pain?

- Relief with defecation may suggest a functional problem, whereas relief with eating may suggest peptic ulcer disease.

Are there any other associated symptoms?

- Fever, diarrhea, and bleeding all suggest an inflammatory or infectious etiology.

III. TESTS AND ASSESSMENTS TO ORDER

- Physical examination, unless the history clearly points to a source
- Laboratory studies
  - Complete blood cell count to rule out infection
  - Chemistry panel for metabolic derangements
  - Amylase and lipase for pancreatitis
  - Urinalysis
  - C-reactive protein and erythrocyte sedimentation rate to rule out active inflammatory disease
- X-rays
  - Flat plate to rule out free air, dilated small bowel or colon, stones, and stool in right colon
  - Right upper quadrant ultrasound for cholelithiasis, biliary dilation, and pancreatic and liver abnormalities

- Computed tomography (CT) scan to rule out abscess, transmural inflammation, pancreatobiliary sources, appendicitis, and vascular abnormalities
- CT enterography and magnetic resonance enterography to rule out active Crohn's disease and look at extraluminal abnormalities
- Endoscopy—rarely helpful unless there are other signs or symptoms of inflammation, such as bleeding or diarrhea

SUGGESTED READINGS

Cohen RD, ed. *Inflammatory Bowel Disease: Diagnosis and Therapeutics*. Totowa, NJ: Humana Press Incorporated; 2003.

Lichtenstein GR, ed. *Clinicians Guide to Inflammatory Bowel Disease*. Thorofare, NJ: SLACK Incorporated; 2003.

Extraintestinal Manifestations

Ellen J. Scherl, MD

Extraintestinal manifestations of IBD occur frequently. Disorders involving practically all organ systems have been reported.

Arthralgias

Arthralgias, or joint pains, in the IBD patient can be due to a variety of conditions, and treatment depends on the underlying etiology.

I. CONDITIONS TO CONSIDER

- Active IBD
- Osteoarthritis
- Tendonitis
- Secondary inflammatory arthritis
- Fracture

Dubinsky M, Friedman S.
Pocket Guide to IBD, Second Edition (pp 19-28).
© 2011 SLACK Incorporated

II. Questions to Ask

Are the joints red, warm, or otherwise "inflamed"?

- Red, warm, inflamed joints could signal true inflammation versus the simple arthralgia that typically accompanies active IBD.

How many joints are involved?

- Involvement of one specific joint could represent either infection or trauma. Involvement of multiple joints suggests either drug reaction or active IBD.

Has the patient had a recent infusion of infliximab?

- Joint complaints following an infusion of infliximab tend to be migratory, polyarticular, and associated with a migratory rash. Patients will usually respond to a Medrol Dosepak (methylprednisolone) or 2 weeks of low-dose prednisone 5 to 10 mg/day.

Does the patient complain of back pain specifically?

- Back pain could signal another inflammatory condition, ankylosing spondylitis, or possible abscess in patients with Crohn's disease. Other considerations are fracture, spinal stenosis, and even kidney stones.

Does the patient complain of hip pain specifically?

- Hip pain could signal fracture or avascular necrosis. (If the patient is currently on steroids or has a history of steroid use in the past, both avascular necrosis and osteoporosis must be considered.)

III. TESTS AND ASSESSMENTS TO ORDER

- X-rays
  - Plain films to rule out skeletal abnormalities
  - Consider computed tomography scan for abscess
  - Consider magnetic resonance imaging to look for other joint and soft-tissue conditions
- Laboratory studies
  - Erythrocyte sedimentation rate and/or C-reactive protein to rule out active inflammation
  - Antinuclear antibody (ANA), anti–double-stranded-DNA antibody, histone antibody, and human leukocyte antigen-B27 to assess for autoimmune arthritis
  - Lyme and Parvovirus titers if patient has any travel history
  - 1,25-hydroxyvitamin D, 25-hydroxyvitamin D, parathyroid hormone, and dual-energy x-ray absorptiometry scan if patient has risk factors for osteoporosis and consider also a celiac panel
- Consider a rheumatology consultation for the multidisciplinary approach to the treatment of many of these joint manifestations, such as ankylosing spondylitis and other potentially debilitating arthropathies

Rash

Certain skin conditions can herald the onset of active disease, and some can run an independent course from any gastrointestinal symptoms.

I. CONDITIONS TO CONSIDER

- Infectious conditions
- Erythema nodosum
- Pyoderma gangrenosum
- Cutaneous Crohn's disease
- Psoriasis/eczema
- Skin cancer

II. QUESTIONS TO ASK

How active are your gastrointestinal symptoms?

- Erythema nodosum and cutaneous Crohn's disease, as well as psoriasis and eczema, are more likely to be active when gastrointestinal symptoms are active.

What does the rash look like?

- A "band" of erythema suggests herpes. Nodules on the extremities may be manifestations of be erythema nodosum, pyoderma gangrenosum, or cutaneous Crohn's disease.
- The lesions of erythema nodosum appear as raised, tender, red or violet subcutaneous nodules usually found on the extensor surfaces of the lower extremities. Biopsy of these lesions,

which show focal panniculitis, is rarely required, and this is usually a clinical diagnosis. Erythema nodosum usually parallels intestinal disease activity and usually responds to treatment of the underlying bowel disease. Severe, refractory lesions or cases that precede bowel symptoms may require systemic corticosteroids.

- Pyoderma gangrenosum begins as a tender papule or pustule that rapidly expands to become a large ulcer with a bluish, undermined border and a necrotic, purulent center. These lesions may be single or multiple, commonly occur on the legs and trunk, and are often exacerbated or caused by trauma. Biopsy of these lesions is not diagnostic and is not recommended, although other causes of cutaneous ulcerations such as vasculitis and infections should be excluded. Treatment for pyoderma gangrenosum may be difficult. Surgical debridement should be avoided because it may cause a pathergic response and worsen the condition. High-dose prednisone or pulse steroids are often-used therapies. Other treatments include topical and intralesional steroids, dapsone, 6-mercaptopurine or azathioprine, and intravenous cyclosporine or infliximab.

- Herpes zoster, or shingles, results from the reactivation of latent varicella-zoster virus and is characterized by a unilateral, painful, vesicular eruption restricted to a dermatome. All immunosuppressed patients should be treated with antiviral therapy (acyclovir or valacyclovir) within 72 hours of onset of herpes zoster, and intravenous acyclovir may be considered for more severe infections including disseminated disease or ophthalmic involvement. Immunosuppressive therapy should be discontinued. Vaccination against varicella-zoster is reasonable for non-immunized patients for whom anti-tumor necrosis factor (TNF) treatment is planned.

Has the patient recently started any new medications?

- A diffuse red rash suggests drug intolerance or allergy.

Does the patient have risk factors for skin cancer?

Has the patient been on steroids?

- Acne can be a side effect of steroid therapy. Steroids predispose patients to infectious agents and poor wound healing.

Has the patient had a recent infusion of infliximab or initiation of another anti-TNF therapy?

- Serious skin reactions such as erythema multiforme, Stevens-Johnson syndrome, and toxic epidermal necrolysis have been reported but are extremely rare. More common are minor infusion reactions. Although the development of eczematous and psoriasiform lesions can be seen, discontinuation of therapy is rarely required.

III. TESTS AND ASSESSMENTS TO ORDER

- Examination of the rash is important, as a biopsy may be necessary.

- In most instances, a history is more important than any tests, and a referral to a dermatologist is prudent if a punch biopsy is needed.

Red Eye

Certain eye conditions can be associated with IBD and should be taken seriously.

I. CONDITIONS TO CONSIDER

- Episcleritis
- Uveitis
- Corneal abrasion or injury
- Infectious conjunctivitis
- Allergic reaction

II. QUESTIONS TO ASK

Is there blurred vision, does the eye hurt, or is there photophobia?

- These symptoms could signal a progressive condition such as episcleritis or uveitis and the patient should be seen by an ophthalmologist, not just an optometrist.
- Episcleritis and uveitis are the most common ocular manifestations of IBD. Episcleritis may be asymptomatic and present as an injection of the ciliary vessels and inflammation of the episcleral tissues without loss of vision. It usually parallels IBD activity. Therapy includes topical corticosteroids. Uveitis manifests with eye pain, blurred vision, photophobia, and headache and

is frequently bilateral. Diagnosis is made on slit-lamp examination revealing inflammation and cells in the anterior chamber. The distinction between episcleritis and uveitis has therapeutic importance because episcleritis often responds to topical anti-inflammatory agents, whereas uveitis typically requires systemic medications and in some cases immunosuppressive drugs.

Is there vision loss?

- Vision loss is an ophthalmologic emergency, and the patient should be seen immediately by an ophthalmologist.

Has the patient been on steroids?

- Cataracts, infections, and retinal detachment can be complications of steroid use, and all patients who are chronically treated with steroids should have regular ophthalmologic examinations.

III. TESTS AND ASSESSMENTS TO ORDER

- The patient with red eye should be seen quickly. If there is eye pain or visual loss, the patient should be seen within hours. Otherwise, the patient should be referred to an ophthalmologist for possible slit-lamp examination.

Suggested Readings

Bernstein CN, Blanchard JF, Rawsthorne P, Yu N. The prevalence of extraintestinal diseases in inflammatory bowel disease: a population-based study. *Am J Gastroenterol.* 2001;96(4):1116-1122.

Bhagat S, Das KM. A shared and unique peptide in the human colon, eye, and joint detected by a monoclonal antibody. *Gastroenterology.* 1994;107(1):103-108.

Borrás-Blasco J, Gracia-Perez A, Nuñez-Cornejo C, et al. Exacerbation of psoriatic skin lesions in a patient with psoriatic arthritis receiving adalimumab. *J Clin Pharm Ther.* 2008;33(3): 321-325.

Calin A. Ankylosing spondylitis. In: Maddison PJ, Isenberg DA, Woo P, Glass DN, eds. *Oxford Textbook of Rheumatology.* Vol. 2. Oxford, United Kingdom: Oxford University Press; 1998;1058-1070.

Cohen JD, Bournerias I, Buffard V, et al. Psoriasis induced by tumor necrosis factor-alpha antagonist therapy: a case series. *J Rheumatol.* 2007;34(2):380-385.

Greenstein AJ, Janowitz HD, Sachar DB. The extra-intestinal complications of Crohn's disease and ulcerative colitis: a study of 700 patients. *Medicine (Baltimore).* 1976;55(5):401-412.

Orchard TR, Dhar A, Simmons JD, Welsh KI, Jewell DP. Phenotype determining genes in the HLA region may determine the presence of uveitis and erythema nodosum (EN) in inflammatory bowel disease. *Gastroenterology.* 2000;118:A869.

Sylvester F. Bone and inflammatory bowel disease. In: Scherl EJ, Dubinsky MC, eds. *The Changing World of Inflammatory Bowel Disease.* Thorofare, NJ: SLACK Incorporated: 2009; 101-116.

Fatigue

Sonia Friedman, MD, FACG

Fatigue is often the most troublesome symptom of IBD. It greatly limits work and social activities and often prevents patients from completing even basic daily routines. It is a major cause of depression in IBD patients. Fatigue stems from a variety of causes, and treating these causes can often make a big difference in a patient's quality of life.

I. CONDITIONS TO CONSIDER

- Active IBD
- Iron-deficiency anemia
- Vitamin B_{12}/folate deficiency
- Malnutrition
- Electrolyte abnormalities
- Chronic pain
- Depression
- Undiagnosed malignancy

Dubinsky M, Friedman S.
Pocket Guide to IBD, Second Edition (pp 29-34).
© 2011 SLACK Incorporated

- Drug reaction
- Adrenal insufficiency
- Unrelated viral infection
- Total parenteral nutrition (TPN) line infection
- Pregnancy
- IBD-related arthritis
- Hypothyroidism
- Use of medications such as prednisone and aza-thioprine (AZA)

II. QUESTIONS TO ASK

How long has the fatigue been present?

- *Several days to a week.* May be due to increased disease activity, drug reaction, electrolyte abnormality, or TPN line infection.
- *Several weeks to months.* May be something more chronic, such as iron/B_{12}/folate deficiency, malnutrition, pregnancy, adrenal insufficiency, IBD-related arthritis, or hypothyroidism.
- *Several months to years.* Harder to correct but must be investigated. Consider chronic pain, depression, and malignancy.

How severe is the fatigue?

- *Mild.* Usually due to mild laboratory abnormality, anemia, mild IBD flare, or unrelated viral infection.
- *Moderate.* May be due to IBD flare, malnutrition, hypothyroidism, or adrenal insufficiency.

- *Severe.* Must be immediately dealt with because it could indicate a life-threatening condition such as a malignancy, severe anemia, or sepsis.

Are there associated symptoms?

- *Abdominal pain/diarrhea.* Can indicate an IBD flare.
- *Weight loss.* Can signal malnutrition, vitamin and mineral deficiencies, or a malignancy.
- *Bleeding.* Can cause anemia.
- *Chronic pain, depression, and inability to leave the house.* Refer for consultation with a pain specialist and/or a psychiatrist.
- *Dizziness/fainting/arthralgias.* Can indicate adrenal insufficiency or can occur while prednisone is being tapered.
- *Arthritis/arthralgias.* Can be due to a serum sickness–like reaction to infliximab or to an autoimmune reaction to infliximab or, more rarely, to adalimumab, certolizumab, or natalizumab.
- *Nausea/vomiting.* Can be due to pregnancy, an IBD flare, or a drug reaction to 6-mercaptopurine (MP)/AZA or methotrexate.
- *Headache.* Can be due to a drug reaction to 6-MP/AZA or, rarely, CNS infection.
- *Fever.* May be caused by infection due to immunocompromised state, or may be due to a drug reaction to 6-MP/AZA.

Are there other behaviors that may be contributing to the fatigue?

- Increased physical or work activity can easily cause fatigue in a chronically ill individual.
- Self-induced vomiting or limiting of food intake due to an eating disorder may cause fatigue. This

is more common than one might think and contributes to malnutrition in certain IBD patients.

- Nonadherence to supplements such as iron, B$_{12}$, folate, or nutritional supplements contributes to anemia and malnutrition.
- Nonadherence to IBD medications may result in IBD flares.
- Certain herbal preparations can cause fatigue. Always examine carefully what the patient is taking. Patients should bring pill bottles and all over-the-counter medications to the office visit.
- Some women feel more fatigued around their menstrual periods and also experience IBD flares during menstruation.

What is the patient's current IBD therapy?

- 6-MP/AZA can cause fatigue as a side effect.
- Infliximab can cause fatigue through several mechanisms. Patients can develop an autoimmune reaction consisting of fatigue/arthralgias/fevers, a positive antinuclear antibody (ANA), and, rarely, anti–double-stranded-DNA antibodies. With long lapses in between infusions, patients can also develop a serum sickness–like reaction consisting of fevers, arthralgias, and fatigue.
- Adalimumab/certolizumab/natalizumab can also cause fatigue by a serum sickness–like reaction, although this is more rare than that occurring with infliximab.
- Prednisone can lead to fatigue. After taking prednisone for as little as 3 months, patients can develop adrenal insufficiency after the prednisone is tapered. Patients tapered to 10 mg or less of prednisone should be tested by either a morning cortisol level or a cortisol stimulation test.

In addition, the process of tapering prednisone itself can cause fatigue and arthralgias.

III. Tests and Assessments to Order

With fatigue that lasts longer than 1 week, the patient should be evaluated. The following tests may be ordered:

- Laboratory studies
  - Complete blood count, vitamin B_{12}, folate, electrolyte levels, albumin, and thyroid-stimulating hormone, which assess for anemia, infection, malnutrition, hypothyroidism, and electrolyte imbalances
  - Morning cortisol level or cortisol stimulation test in appropriate patients
  - Blood, urine, and stool cultures in febrile patients or in immunosuppressed patients who are moderately to severely fatigued to rule out an occult infection
  - Urine or serum human chorionic gonadotropin in women of childbearing age
  - ANA and anti–double-stranded-DNA for patients on infliximab
- Calorie counts and consultation with a nutritionist in appropriate patients
- Psychiatric evaluation for patients with depression or eating disorders
- Pain specialist evaluation for patients with chronic pain
- Physical examination assessing for tachycardia, hypotension, lymphadenopathy, thyromegaly, abdominal mass, and blood on rectal examination
- Back and spine x-rays for certain patients with joint complaints

Suggested Readings

Graff LA, Vincent N, Walker JR, et al. A population-based study of fatigue and sleep difficulties in inflammatory bowel disease [published online ahead of print December 22, 2010]. *Inflamm Bowel Dis.* doi:10.1002/ibd.21580.

Jelsness-Jørgensen LP, Bernklev T, Henriksen M, Torp R, Moum BA. Chronic fatigue is more prevalent in patients with inflammatory bowel disease than in healthy controls [published online ahead of print November 8, 2010]. *Inflamm Bowel Dis.* doi:10.1002/ibd.21530.

Marcus SB, Strople JA, Neighbors K, et al. Fatigue and health-related quality of life in pediatric inflammatory bowel disease. *Clin Gastroenterol Hepatol.* 2009;7(5):554-561.

Fever

Sonia Friedman, MD, FACG

Fever in IBD can signal disease activity, an IBD complication, or a drug reaction. It can range from a low-grade fever responsive to acetaminophen to high fevers and shaking chills that require hospitalization. Fever in IBD has a long list of causes, and only careful questioning and examination will elucidate the problem.

I. CONDITIONS TO CONSIDER

- Active IBD
- Intra-abdominal perforation
- Intra-abdominal abscess
- Drug reaction
- Postoperative fever
- Total parenteral nutrition (TPN) line infection
- Unrelated viral or bacterial infection
- Infection due to immunosuppression
- Deep venous thrombosis
- Kidney stone

Dubinsky M, Friedman S.
Pocket Guide to IBD, Second Edition (pp 35-40).
© 2011 SLACK Incorporated

- A medical condition that may be related to IBD (eg, cholecystitis/cholangitis/pancreatitis)
- A medical condition that is not necessarily related to IBD (eg, appendicitis, diverticulitis, myocardial infarction, cerebrovascular accident, hematologic malignancy)

II. QUESTIONS TO ASK

How high is the fever?

- *Low-grade fever.* May be postoperative, caused by increased IBD activity, or due to a drug reaction. Will abate when the precipitant is treated or removed.
- *High-grade fever.* May be caused by something more serious, such as a bowel perforation or an abscess. Usually requires at least an emergency room visit.

How long has the fever lasted?

- *A day or two.* Can be due to increased IBD activity or any other condition that has just started. Will require removal of precipitant and/or correlation with other symptoms.
- *Longer than a couple of days.* Needs evaluation and further testing.

What other symptoms are associated with the fever?

- *Abdominal pain.* Worry about abscess or perforation.
- *Diarrhea.* Worry about increased IBD activity.
- *Back pain.* Worry about kidney stone or kidney infection.

- *Right upper quadrant/epigastric pain.* Worry about biliary/pancreatic complication.
- *Chest pain.* Worry about myocardial infarction, pulmonary embolism, bronchitis, and pneumonia.
- *Upper respiratory symptoms.* Worry about common cold or sinusitis.
- *Postoperative fever.* If persistent, needs thorough evaluation.
- *Asymmetric leg swelling.* Worry about deep venous thrombosis.
- *Abnormal complete blood cell count.* Worry about infection or malignancy.

Are there other behaviors that might be contributing to the fever?

- Increased physical activity, when combined with diarrhea, can cause dehydration which may cause a fever.
- Nonsteroidal anti-inflammatory use can trigger bowel activity and thus cause a fever.
- Antibiotic use can trigger bowel activity and thus cause a fever.
- Over-the-counter preparation use may rarely cause a fever due to a drug reaction.
- In ulcerative colitis, symptoms can flare when patients stop smoking, and in Crohn's disease, smoking can increase the severity of illness.

What is the patient's current IBD therapy?

- Sulfasalazine can cause a drug-induced fever in up to 25% to 30% of patients due to the sulfapyridine component of the drug.
- 6-mercaptopurine (6-MP)/azathioprine (AZA) can cause a drug-induced fever in up to 5%

of patients and can cause pancreatitis in up to 3% to 4% of patients. The pancreatitis usually occurs within the first month of therapy and is reversible when the drug is stopped. If either 6-MP or AZA is restarted, the pancreatitis will always recur. 6-MP/AZA can also cause a febrile neutropenia if the patient is homozygous for the thiopurine methyltransferase (TPMT) allele or if the dose is too high in patients with the other 2 TPMT genotypes. It is now common practice to measure TPMT genotype/phenotype at the start of 6-MP/AZA therapy and to check a complete blood cell count (CBC) every 2 weeks after a dose change for at least 4 weeks and every 2 months thereafter.

- 6-MP/AZA + 5-aminosalicylate agents rarely can cause a febrile neutropenia.
- 6-MP/AZA + allopurinol can cause a profound leukopenia.
- With infliximab therapy, fevers can be associated with an infusion reaction or can be due to infection. Fevers can also be associated with a serum sickness–like reaction due to long periods in between infliximab doses.
- Adalimumab/certolizumab can also cause fever by a serum sickness–like reaction, although this is more rare than with infliximab.
- With natalizumab therapy, fevers can be caused by an infusion reaction, an infection, or a serum sickness–like reaction.
- Immunosuppression   (6-MP/AZA/infliximab/ methotrexate, cyclosporine/prednisone) can predispose patients to various infections such as Epstein-Barr virus, histoplasmosis, herpetic infection, cytomegalovirus colitis, bacterial sepsis, disseminated tuberculosis.

- Patients with a TPN line may acquire a line infection. If fever develops in these patients, peripheral and central line blood cultures should be obtained immediately.

III. Tests and Assessments to Order

Often, patients who present with fever will need a thorough evaluation. Depending on the patient's symptoms, the following tests should be performed.

- Laboratory studies
  - CBC with differential to help diagnose infection, leukopenia, malignancy, and anemia
  - Electrolyte panel to assess for dehydration
  - Urinalysis to look for infection or blood indicating a kidney stone
  - Stool studies—always check bacterial cultures, *Clostridium difficile* toxin, *Giardia* antigen if patient has increased gas and bloating and has done some outdoor travel, and ova and parasites if patient is on immunosuppressive agents
  - Peripheral and line blood cultures, if the patient has a central line, to rule out sepsis
- Physical examination—take patient's temperature, look for costovertebral angle or abdominal tenderness, listen for pneumonia, check for tachycardia and hypotension, look for asymmetric leg swelling
- Computed tomography scan of the abdomen and pelvis to rule out a perforation, abscess, kidney stone, and biliary or pancreatic complication

SUGGESTED READINGS

Kornbluth A, Sachar DB; Practice Parameters Committee of the American College of Gastroenterology. Ulcerative colitis practice guidelines in adults: American College Of Gastroenterology, Practice Parameters Committee. *Am J Gastroenterol.* 2010;105(3):501-523.

Lichtenstein GR, Hanauer SB, Sandborn WJ; Practice Parameters Committee of American College of Gastroenterology. Management of Crohn's disease in adults. *Am J Gastroenterol.* 2009;104(2):465-483.

Diarrhea

Kim L. Isaacs, MD, PhD

Diarrhea is one of the common symptoms indicating a flare of disease activity in IBD. Diarrhea associated with IBD has many potential etiologies, running the spectrum from medication side effect to superimposed infection (Table 7-1).

I. CONDITIONS TO CONSIDER

- Active IBD
- *Clostridium difficile* infection
- Cytomegalovirus infection
- Medication side effect
- Small bowel bacterial overgrowth
- Bile acid diarrhea
- Irritable bowel syndrome
- Infectious gastroenteritis
- Lactose intolerance
- Hyperthyroidism
- Celiac disease (gluten-sensitive enteropathy)

Dubinsky M, Friedman S.
Pocket Guide to IBD, Second Edition (pp 41-50).
© 2011 SLACK Incorporated

Chapter 7

Table 7-1. Noninfectious Diarrhea in the Patient With IBD

Disease Process	Features	Tests	Treatment
Irritable bowel syndrome	May coexist with IBD Nonbloody diarrhea No inflammatory markers May be triggered by food intake Associated cramping	Exclude active IBD and other causes of diarrhea	Fiber antispasmodics
Lactose intolerance	Made worse with dairy products Associated gas and cramping	Hydrogen breath test using lactose ingestion	Avoid lactose-containing products; products are available with lactase to aid in processing of lactose.
Bile salt malabsorption	Appropriate setting— seen in patients with terminal ileal resection or inflammation May also be seen in patients with cholecystectomy	SeHCAT (selenium-75-homocholic acid taurine) testing → not available in United States—diagnosis made by looking at clinical presentation and response to therapy	Use of a bile salt binder such as cholestyramine

(continued)

Table 7-1. Noninfectious Diarrhea in the Patient With IBD (continued)

Disease Process	Features	Tests	Treatment
Gluten-sensitive enteropathy (celiac disease, sprue)	Malabsorptive process Made worse with gluten-containing diet	Anti-tissue transglutaminase AB (anti-TTG) Antiendomysial antibody Human leukocyte antigen testing—HLA-DQ2, HLA-DQ8 Upper endoscopy with biopsy on a gluten-containing diet	Gluten-free diet
Small bowel bacterial overgrowth	May be associated with small bowel strictures, ileocecal valve resection, poor small bowel motility Patients may complain of bloating and passage of foul-smelling gas per rectum	Hydrogen breath test	Antibiotic therapy—antibiotics that have been used include tetracycline, ciprofloxacin, metronidazole, and rifaximin

(continued)

Table 7-1. Noninfectious Diarrhea in the Patient With IBD (continued)

Disease Process	Features	Tests	Treatment
Malabsorptive diarrhea	May be due to extensive small bowel resection or small bowel disease Large-volume diarrhea Decreased diarrhea with fasting Stools tend to float, or fat is seen in the toilet water	Spot fecal fat 72-hour quantitative fat Stool volume measurements with fasting and nonfasting	Low-fat diet Polymeric liquid diet supplements

II. QUESTIONS TO ASK

What is the nature of the diarrhea?

- *Small volume, bloody, with tenesmus.* Suggests active rectal inflammation.
- *Large volume, nonbloody.* Can be seen in small intestinal disease such as recurrent Crohn's disease and infectious enteritis.
- *Blood mixed in with diarrhea.* Suggests an active colitic process.
- *Diarrhea stops with fasting.* In diarrhea due to malabsorption, stool volume will decrease with fasting.
- *Diarrhea fluctuates with intermittent constipation.* Consider irritable bowel syndrome.

How do current bowel habits compare to baseline stool frequency, consistency, and volume? How did the diarrhea start?

- Many patients with IBD have altered baseline bowel habits due to disease activity, prior surgeries, and medical therapy.
- Increased diarrhea associated with a flare in disease activity is typically insidious in onset.
- Acute onset of diarrhea in an otherwise stable baseline is suggestive of an infectious process.

What is the patient's current medication history?

- Check to see if the patient has recently changed IBD medications or has had other non-IBD medications added to regimen.
- Of all of the IBD medications commonly used, 5-aminosalicylates may be associated with worsening diarrhea. Osalazine may cause a secretory diarrhea in up to 20% of patients with initiation of therapy.
- In patients on chronic immunosuppressive therapies such as 6-mercaptopurine, azathioprine, methotrexate, and/or maintenance anti-tumor necrosis factor therapy, there is a risk of opportunistic infections that may cause diarrhea, such as cytomegalovirus infection.
- Nonsteroidal anti-inflammatories may be associated with IBD flares and in addition may cause diarrhea independently as a side effect.
- Proton pump inhibitors such as omeprazole may be associated with diarrhea.
- Recent antibiotic use raises the question of *C difficile* infection. Of note, *C difficile* infection can also occur in the absence of antibiotic exposure and is seen with increasing frequency in the IBD population.

Has the patient had any gastrointestinal surgery?

- Resection of the terminal ileum may lead to bile acid malabsorption and a subsequent secretory diarrhea related to the bile acids.
- Patients who have had more than 100 cm of small bowel resected are at risk for fat and nutrient malabsorption due to decreased surface area of the bowel.

Has the patient ever had a bowel stricture?

- Stricturing disease may lead to small bowel bacterial overgrowth with signs of diarrhea, abdominal bloating, and excessive gas per rectum.

Is the diarrhea associated with any type of food intake?

- Acquired carbohydrate malabsorption may occur with disruption of the brush border enzymes during active inflammation.
- Celiac disease (sprue) can coexist with Crohn's disease, and symptoms may be exacerbated by gluten-containing products.
- Lactose intolerance may coexist with IBD. Certain sugar substitutes such as sorbitol may produce an osmotic diarrhea.

Is the diarrhea associated with the patient's menstrual cycle?

- Hormonal changes during different points of the menstrual cycle may be associated with increased bowel activity and diarrhea.

III. TESTS AND ASSESSMENTS TO ORDER

If the diarrhea is mild, supportive therapy can be used, but if the diarrhea is persistent, evaluation will likely be required. Evaluation can be tailored in part to the suspected cause or consequence of the diarrhea.

- Laboratory studies
  - *Complete cell blood count.* In acute inflammation or active inflammatory disease, there may be an elevated white blood cell count, elevated platelet count, and anemia.
  - *Electrolyte panel.* Profuse watery diarrhea may lead to dehydration and electrolyte depletion, which will need replacement. Magnesium depletion is common in patients with short bowel syndrome.
  - *Zinc level.* Zinc deficiency is not uncommon in IBD and may lead to diarrhea, which, in turn, leads to increased difficulties with zinc depletion.
  - Celiac disease serology (anti-tissue transglutaminase and/or antiendomysial antibodies).
  - *Stool studies.*
    - Check for *C difficile* toxin, bacterial screen, and parasites. *Giardia* may be superimposed on underlying IBD.
    - Check a stool white blood cell count. A nonelevated count would argue against an acute infectious colitis.
    - If the stool is liquid, stool electrolytes (sodium and potassium) can be assessed to delineate a secretory from a malabsorptive diarrheal process.
    - A spot fecal fat can be checked to look grossly for fat malabsorption.
    - Fecal calprotectin or fecal lactoferrin may help delineate an inflammatory diarrhea from irritable bowel syndrome–associated diarrhea.
- *Physical examination.* Look for signs of dehydration, such as dry mucous membranes, decreased axillary sweat, and poor skin turgor. On abdominal examination, tenderness suggests active

inflammation. Tenderness would be less likely with a bile acid diarrhea or diarrhea secondary to bacterial overgrowth or lactose intolerance.
- *Flexible sigmoidoscopy.* Active inflammation and pseudomembranes can be identified visually. Biopsies should be performed to rule out superimposed cytomegalovirus colitis. This can be done by polymerase chain reaction analysis, routine histology, and immunohistochemistry of the biopsy specimens. Ruling out CMV is especially important in patients who are on chronic immunosuppressive agents.
- Hydrogen breath test to assist in diagnosing bacterial overgrowth and lactose intolerance.

Suggested Readings

Baldi F, Bianco M, et al. Focus on acute diarrhoeal disease. *World J Gastroenterol.* 2009;15(27):3341-3348.

Caccaro R, D'Incá R, et al. Clinical utility of calprotectin and lactoferrin as markers of inflammation in patients with inflammatory bowel disease. *Expert Rev Clin Immunol.* 2010;6(4): 551-558.

Wingate D, Phillips S, et al. Guidelines for adults on self-medication for the treatment of acute diarrhoea. *Aliment Pharmacol Ther.* 2001;15(6):773-782.

Nausea

Debra J. Helper, MD

Within the context of IBD, nausea can be due to any of a number of causes seen in individuals without IBD or it may be due to a recurrence of the disease, a complication of the disease, or a side effect of therapy.

I. CONDITIONS TO CONSIDER

- Gastroesophageal reflux disease or peptic disease
- Small bowel or gastric outlet obstruction due to stricture or adhesions
- Active IBD, especially Crohn's disease of the upper gastrointestinal (GI) tract
- Medication side effect
- Adrenal insufficiency (in patients previously on chronic corticosteroid therapy)
- Liver disease (hepatitis related to medication, infection, or malignancy)
- Gallbladder disease

Dubinsky M, Friedman S.
Pocket Guide to IBD, Second Edition (pp 51-56).
© 2011 SLACK Incorporated

- Central nervous system causes
- Pancreatic disease

II. QUESTIONS TO ASK

Is the nausea persistent or does it occur during only part of the day?

- Morning nausea could be related to medications, but do not forget about the possibility of pregnancy. Many women with IBD may have irregular periods and may not know that they are pregnant.

How long has the patient been nauseated?

- A day suggests an acute process, whereas days to weeks could signal worsening disease or medication reaction.

Is the patient also vomiting?

- Vomiting along with nausea may suggest obstruction and should prompt assessment for more acute conditions.

What is the nature of the emesis?

- Old food suggests gastric outlet obstruction; blood suggests ulcerative disease, bleeding from a complication such as primary sclerosing cholangitis with variceal bleeding, or Crohn's disease of the proximal small bowel.

Is the nausea related to food?

- Nausea that is improved with food may signal peptic ulcer disease. Nausea that is not relieved with food intake, or made worse, may be IBD or medication related.

Is there associated abdominal pain?

- Crampy abdominal pain suggests active small bowel disease, sharp pain radiating through to the back can be a sign of pancreatitis, colicky right upper quadrant pain is more consistent with a biliary source, burning epigastric pain may be caused by ulcer or gastroesophageal reflux, and severe colicky abdominal pain suggests obstruction.

Is the patient's abdomen distended?

- Significant abdominal distention is worrisome for distal obstruction, whereas proximal small bowel or gastric outlet obstruction may occur without significant distention but can cause a great deal of nausea. Severe colicky pain with distention and vomiting suggests high-grade obstruction and requires immediate evaluation.

What medications and supplements is the patient currently taking?

- Many IBD therapies are notorious for nausea as a side effect. They include (but are not limited to) iron, metronidazole, azathioprine/6-mercaptopurine (6-MP) (with or without side effects of pancreatitis or hepatitis), sulfasalazine, methotrexate, and narcotics (causing either central nausea or nausea due to decreased intestinal motility). If the nausea is related to azathioprine, switching to 6-MP may help. If the patient develops pancreatitis or fever related to 6-MP, this class of drugs should be stopped altogether. Nausea/vomiting is usually an isolated symptom and may be temporally related to the ingestion of the medication.

III. ACTIONS TO TAKE/TESTS AND ASSESSMENTS TO ORDER

- If symptoms are mild, consider a trial of a proton pump inhibitor. Metoclopramide may be useful if dysmotility is suspected but is contraindicated if there is a possibility of obstruction.
- If symptoms are temporally associated with administration of a medication, adjust or hold the medication to see if the nausea abates. In the case of metronidazole, an acceptable alternative might be used, or a trial of the enteric coated (375-mg pill) form can be used. Similarly with sulfasalazine, the EN-tab formulation may be better tolerated. Alternatively, mesalamine products can be substituted at equivalent doses, as they are less likely to cause nausea since they lack the sulfapyridine moiety present in sulfasalazine. Narcotic use should be minimized. Splitting the daily dose of azathioprine or 6-MP and taking with food, or before bedtime, may alleviate nausea. Administering additional folic acid may improve nausea due to methotrexate.
- If patients are unable to keep down any fluids, have them go to the emergency room, where they can be evaluated for physical findings of

obstruction and have plain films of the abdomen (obstructive series) performed. If suspicion is strong for obstruction but there is lack of clear evidence on the plain films, consider an abdominal computed tomography scan to evaluate for fluid-filled loops of bowel or a closed-loop obstruction due to adhesion.

- Laboratory studies
  - Amylase, lipase, and other liver enzymes
  - Complete blood cell count
  - Inflammatory markers, such as C-reactive protein and erythrocyte sedimentation rate
  - Fasting morning cortisol, cosyntropin stimulation test (as indicated if adrenal insufficiency is suspected)
  - Electrolyte panel, including magnesium and calcium (derangements may cause dysmotility and exacerbate nausea in patients with vomiting and/or diarrhea)
- Right upper quadrant ultrasound to help document cholecystitis and pancreatic disease.
- Upper GI endoscopy to evaluate for active upper GI tract Crohn's disease, peptic ulcer disease, and gastric outlet or proximal small bowel obstruction, which may be relieved by endoscopic dilation and/or steroid injection.
- Enteroclysis or video capsule endoscopy (VCE). These tests may need to be performed to clearly demonstrate active small bowel disease as the source of nausea. VCE is contraindicated in patients suspected of having obstruction and should be performed in patients with IBD only after radiographic small bowel imaging reveals no evidence of narrowing.
- Magnetic resonance imaging of the brain and brainstem if a central source is considered a possibility.

Suggested Readings

Riello L, Talbotec C, Garnier-Lengliné H, et al. Tolerance and efficacy of azathioprine in pediatric Crohn's disease [published online ahead of print January 13, 2011]. *Inflamm Bowel Dis*. doi:10.1002/ibd.21612.

Shah B, Tinsley A, Ullman T. Quality of care in inflammatory bowel disease [published online ahead of print November 16, 2010]. *Curr Gastroenterol Rep*. doi:10.1007/s11894-010-0155-7.

Siegel CA. Review article: explaining risks of inflammatory bowel disease therapy to patients. *Aliment Pharmacol Ther*. 2011;33(1):23-32.

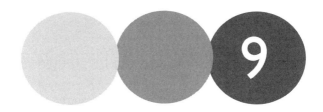

Rectal Bleeding

Sunanda V. Kane, MD, MSPH, FACG, FACP, AGAF

Rectal bleeding is one of the key symptoms that signals possible disease activity. However, bleeding as an individual symptom runs a full spectrum from simple hemorrhoids to life-threatening hemorrhage. It is the careful consideration of the accompanying symptoms that helps appropriately triage the patient.

I. CONDITIONS TO CONSIDER

- Active IBD
- Fistula bleeding
- Hemorrhoids/fissure
- Gynecologic bleeding
- Concurrent colitis
- Malignancy
- Infections
- Polyps

Dubinsky M, Friedman S.
Pocket Guide to IBD, Second Edition (pp 57-60).
© 2011 SLACK Incorporated

II. Questions to Ask

What is the nature of the bleeding?

- *Drops of fresh blood on the toilet paper or in the toilet bowl.* Suggests hemorrhoids or other anal canal abnormalities, such as anal fissure.
- *Mixed in stool.* Suggests possible active colitis or ileitis. Polyps should also be considered.
- *Clots.* May signal active bleeding.
- *Spontaneous bleeding.* Blood seen with or without bowel movements may signal very active disease.

How long has the bleeding been going on?

- Patients may wait for a significant amount of time before calling the office. The longer the bleeding has been going on, the more time it will take to resolve.

Are there associated symptoms?

- *Rectal pain.* This can be associated with Crohn's disease, ulcerative colitis (UC), or an anal fissure/ulcer.
- *Urgency.* This signals inflammation in the rectum.
- *Straining.* Very active left-sided disease may cause a relative constipation on the right side of the colon and result in straining. This also can be associated with rectal inflammation.
- *Diarrhea.* This may signal active disease or another concurrent colitis.

Are there other behaviors that may be contributing to the problem?

- Estimates suggest that regular use of nonsteroidal anti-inflammatory drugs is associated with a 30% risk of precipitating a flare of IBD symptoms.
- Certain antibiotics, particularly the penicillin-based ones, can cause gastrointestinal symptoms as well as *Clostridium difficile* infection.
- In patients with UC, smoking cessation can precipitate a flare; in patients with Crohn's disease, continued smoking can potentiate disease activity.
- Women may notice a pattern of more active symptoms related to their menstrual cycle.

What is the patient's current IBD therapy?

- Patients who stop taking their maintenance medications are likely to have flares. Be mindful that some patients may be taking a fraction of what you may think they are taking. Patients who have recently been started on a 5-aminosalicylate compound may experience hypersensitivity or increased bleeding. Hypersensitivity can occur in up to 7% of patients who are prescribed this class of medicines. In women, ask about any change in oral contraceptive preparations, as this may lead to a disease flare.
- Some patients will not admit to taking supplements or over-the-counter therapies. Nonsteroidal anti-inflammatories as well as compounds containing magnesium may cause diarrhea and precipitate a flare.
- Many herbal compounds have unknown toxicities and must be considered in the differential.

III. Tests and Assessments to Order

- Laboratory studies
  - *Complete blood cell count (CBC)*. Comparison with a baseline CBC will help tell the chronicity and/or severity of the bleeding.
  - *Stool studies*. Do not waste time checking fecal leukocytes, since they will be present if there is visible blood. Remember to check for *C difficile* toxin as well as other appropriate bacterial cultures depending on the patient's history. Patients do not necessarily need to have a history of antibiotic use to have *C difficile* colitis.
- *Physical examination*. Check for pallor, tachycardia, skin turgor, and overall appearance. A rectal exam is imperative.
- *Flexible sigmoidoscopy*. In addition to conducting an endoscopic evaluation, be sure to get biopsies if there is active disease to rule out cytomegalovirus colitis.
- A colonoscopy can be performed to rule out transverse or right colon inflammation and also non–IBD-related causes of bleeding such as arteriovenous malformations and diverticular bleeding.

Suggested Readings

Cohen RD, ed. *Inflammatory Bowel Disease: Diagnosis and Therapeutics*. Totowa, NJ: Humana Press Incorporated; 2003.

Lichtenstein GR, ed. *Clinicians Guide to Inflammatory Bowel Disease*. Thorofare, NJ: SLACK Incorporated; 2003.

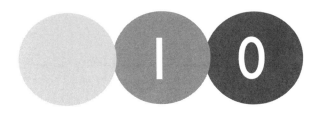

Anorectal Pain

Sara N. Horst, MD and David A. Schwartz, MD

Anorectal pain in a patient with IBD can be caused by very different disease entities. Given that perianal manifestations of Crohn's disease such as fistulas can be extremely difficult to treat, it is important to accurately define the extent of disease and to develop a timely diagnostic and treatment strategy.

I. CONDITIONS TO CONSIDER

- Anal skin tag
- Anal ulcer
- Anal fissure
- Perianal fistula
- Rectovaginal or rectovesicular fistula
- Perianal abscess
- Anorectal stricture
- Anorectal cancer
- Proctalgia fugax

Dubinsky M, Friedman S.
Pocket Guide to IBD, Second Edition (pp 61-66).
© 2011 SLACK Incorporated

II. Questions to Ask

What is the nature of the pain, and when does the pain occur?

- *Pain with defecation.* This may imply disease confined to the anal region, such as an anal ulcer, perianal abscess, or anal fissure. Unlike non-Crohn's–related fissures, Crohn's-related anal fissures can often be asymptomatic. Anal skin tags are common and most often painless.
- *Pain with sitting.* Patients with perirectal abscesses may have difficulty sitting in certain positions.
- *Nonlocalized, continuous pain.* A fistula or abscess can present with nonspecific lower abdominal/rectal pain.
- *Spontaneous pain, lasting only a few seconds to minutes in a patient without bowel symptoms.* Functional pain disorders such as proctalgia fugax should be considered.

Are there associated symptoms?

- *Perianal ulcer or drainage.* Can be a manifestation of Crohn's disease. It is important to ask about this symptom, as patients may not realize that it may be associated with IBD.
- *Fevers/chills.* Could suggest abscess or active disease.
- *Diarrhea.* Suggests active Crohn's disease.
- *Urgency.* Usually indicates active proctitis.
- *Rectal bleeding.* May be secondary to anal fissures, anal ulcers, or active disease.
- *Constipation.* Rarely, can be caused by a stricture or anorectal cancer. Occasionally, patients with severe proctitis will have significant constipation.

- *Frequent urinary tract infections or cloudy urine.* Could imply the presence of a rectovaginal (or rectovesicular) fistula.
- *Passage of air or stool through the vagina, or pain with intercourse.* Could imply the presence of a rectovaginal fistula.

Is there a history of previous IBD, and what is its nature and location?

- *Distal colitis.* Patients with a history of distal colonic Crohn's disease, especially with involvement of the rectum, are much more likely to develop perianal fistulas or abscesses compared to those whose disease is isolated to the ileum.
- *History of fistulas or abscesses.* Fistulas can be very difficult to completely heal, and patients with a history of fistula are at increased risk of recurrence or incomplete healing.

III. TESTS AND ASSESSMENTS TO ORDER

- *Physical examination.* Careful examination of the perianal area is important, as this can aid in diagnosis and will often also determine the next evaluation strategy, especially if fistulizing Crohn's disease is suspected.
  - When secondary to Crohn's disease, anal fissures (mucosal tears or ulcers) can be in unusual locations (eg, lateral), and multiple fissures can be present.
  - Erythema, swelling, or fluctuance suggests perianal abscess and/or fistula.
  - Perianal ulcer or draining lesion suggests perianal abscess and/or fistula.

- ○ Anorectal stricture, usually from previous perianal disease, could increase the likelihood of abscess or fistula.
- ○ If the examination is unrevealing, consider functional disorder or disease not visible on physical examination, such as distal colonic disease.
- *Other tests.* Accurate determination of the extent of disease is vital for delineating an appropriate treatment plan (Figure 10-1). If a patient has a perianal abscess or severe fistulizing disease, gastroenterologists and surgeons often must work together to obtain the best outcomes.
  - ○ *Endoscopy.* It is important to know if the patient has active proctitis, as the presence of proctitis increases the likelihood of perianal disease and can alter the treatment strategies for any fistulas that are present.
  - ○ If perianal fistula or abscess is suspected, several options are available to further define the perianal disease after endoscopy. A combination of pelvic magnetic resonance imaging (MRI) or rectal endoscopic ultrasonography (EUS) with examination under anesthesia (EUA) has been shown to accurately define the perianal disease. This combination approach may be the most useful diagnostic strategy.
    - ➢ Rectal EUS requires a physician with expertise in this area but has been shown to be very sensitive and specific.
    - ➢ Pelvic MRI is a sensitive test, especially if a dedicated pelvic coil is used.
    - ➢ EUA is an advantageous strategy, as the surgeon can provide therapy as well as diagnosis if needed. May be best used after MRI or rectal EUS is performed.

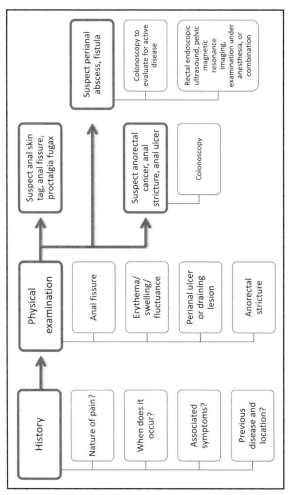

Figure 10-1. Algorithm for evaluating patients with IBD and anorectal pain.

SUGGESTED READINGS

Ingle SB, Loftus EV, Jr. The natural history of perianal Crohn's disease. *Dig Liver Dis.* 2007;39(10):963-969.

Schwartz DA, Wiersema MJ, Dudiak KM, et al. A comparison of endoscopic ultrasound, magnetic resonance imaging, and exam under anesthesia for evaluation of Crohn's perianal fistulas. *Gastroenterology.* 2001;121(5):1064-1072.

Section III

MEDICATIONS AND
OTHER THERAPIES

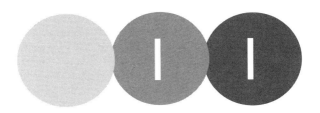

Anti-Tumor Necrosis Factor Therapy and Management

Kim L. Isaacs, MD, PhD

Currently, 3 anti-tumor necrosis factor (TNF) therapies are available for use in IBD. These are infliximab, adalimumab, and certolizumab. The pretreatment evaluation protocol is similar for each of these anti-TNF agents. However, a few differences in management of these therapies exist due to the different routes and timing of administration of the available anti-TNF agents.

Infliximab, Adalimumab, and Certolizumab

I. Prior to Initiating Therapy

- Perform a tuberculosis skin test (purified protein derivative [PPD]) to rule out latent tuberculosis

Dubinsky M, Friedman S.
Pocket Guide to IBD, Second Edition (pp 69-74).
© 2011 SLACK Incorporated

(TB). If the potential risk of prior TB exposure is high and the patient is likely to be anergic, consider QuantiFERONR-TB Gold (QFT-G) assay, which is a whole blood assay based on gamma-interferon production, and a chest x-ray to document lack of evidence for TB. Also perform a chest x-ray in patients who are at high risk for fungal disease.

- Review the patient's immunomodulator history (6-mercaptopurine/azathioprine).
  - Is the patient on an immunomodulator?
  - If not, should an immunomodulator be initated?
  - If yes, should it be continued?
  - Has there been an adverse reaction to immunomodulators in the past?
- Review the patient's immunization history, and immunize when appropriate.
- Review with the patient the risks of therapy and what to look for in terms of risks and side effects, both short and long term.
- Review with the patient the concepts of induction and maintenance therapy.

Infliximab

I. Dosing

- Administration is intravenous (IV).
- Initial dosing is 5 mg/kg body weight at 0, 2, and 6 weeks.
- Decide whether premedication is required. Premedication strategies may include an antihistamine, acetaminophen, and/or a steroid. There are some data that premedication with a steroid prior to infusion may decrease anti-infliximab antibody titer in a patient who is not on other immunosuppressants.

- If induction dosing is successful, maintenance dosing is initiated at 5mg/kg every 8 weeks and adjusted depending on response.
- Patient education information is available at www.remicade.com.

II. In the Event of Reaction During the Infusion

- Shut off the infusion.
- Assess the patient's vital signs and whether there is a rash, wheezing, or swelling to indicate an impending serious problem.
- If the symptoms are mild:
  - Administer diphenhydramine 50 mg IV along with acetaminophen 650 mg orally and consider steroids. If IV diphenhydramine is given, the patient will need to be driven home due to central nervous system effects.
  - If the patient develops rigors, meperidine 25 to 50 mg administered subcutaneously or IV will help, although the patient will have to be accompanied home if narcotics are given.
  - Discuss with the patient the risks and benefits of continuing treatment both acutely and long term.
  - If the patient is interested in continuing the therapy and is stable to do so, restart the infusion at a slower rate after the symptoms have abated.
- If the reaction is severe, the infusion should not be restarted, and if the patient is not responding to supportive therapy, he or she may need to be transported to the emergency department for further supportive management for anaphylaxis.
- Document the specifics of the reaction for future reference.

- Follow up with the patient in the next few days to assess the efficacy of the infliximab infusion.
- Premedicate the patient prior to subsequent infusions. Common combinations include acetaminophen with a nonsedating antihistamine, such as cetirizine or loratadine. Consider premedication with steroids.

III. DELAYED HYPERSENSITIVITY

- The patient will likely call 6 to 10 days following an infusion with complaints of malaise, fever, diffuse arthralgias, and myalgias.
- If the symptoms are mild (ie, the patient is ambulatory but uncomfortable), give acetaminophen as required.
- If the symptoms are moderate, give steroids 20 to 40 mg/day until the symptoms abate (usually 3 to 4 days), then taper rapidly.
- If the symptoms are severe (ie, the patient is unable to walk without assistance), consider hospitalization for IV fluids and steroids.
- If considering retreatment with infliximab, pretreatment with steroids, histamine blockers, and acetaminophen is imperative. With other anti-TNF options available, it would be best to avoid retreatment with infliximab. Patients with a delayed hypersensitivity reaction are also more likely to have an attenuated response to the infliximab.
- Consider ordering infliximab levels and levels of antibodies to infliximab. If no infliximab is present but antibodies are present and greater than 8 µg/mL, the patient may not be a good candidate for retreatment, and switching to a different anti-TNF therapy would be preferable.

Determination of infliximab levels and antibodies is best done as a trough, immediately prior to the next scheduled infusion.

Adalimumab

I. DOSING

- Administration is subcutaneous (40 mg per syringe or pen).
- Loading dose is 160 mg (4 prefilled syringes or pens) at week 0 and 80 mg (2 syringes or pens) at week 2.
- Food and Drug Administration (FDA)–approved maintenance dosing is 40 mg every 2 weeks.
- Premedication is not routinely recommended.

II. SPECIAL CONSIDERATIONS

- Patients who have trouble with the pen method of injection due to injection site discomfort may do better with the prefilled syringe, where the drug can be administered more slowly.
- Icing the injection site prior to injection may decrease injection site reactions.
- If there is a loss of efficacy of the adalimumab, there may be antibody production to the drug, and alteration of the frequency of administration (ie, weekly dosing) may be beneficial.
- Patient education material is available at www.humira.com.

Certolizumab

I. DOSING

- Administration is subcutaneous.

- Each syringe contains 200 mg of certolizumab.
- Loading dose is 400 mg at week 0 and 400 mg at weeks 2 and 4.
- FDA-approved maintenance dosing is 400 mg every 4 weeks.
- Premedication is not routinely recommended.

II. Special Considerations

- Dosing formulations currently available include a prefilled syringe and a lyophilized powder for reconstitution.
- The drug should be at room temperature prior to injection.
- For the 400-mg dose, 2 200-mg injections are given at separate sites.
- Patient education material is available at www.cimzia.com.

Suggested Readings

Connell W, Andrews J, Brown S, et al. Practical guidelines for treating inflammatory bowel disease safely with anti-tumour necrosis factor therapy in Australia. *Intern Med J*. 2010;40(2): 139-149.

Culver E, Travis S. How to manage the infectious risk under anti-TNF in inflammatory bowel disease. *Curr Drug Targets*. 2010;11(2):198-218.

Hoentjen F, van Bodegraven A. Safety of anti-tumor necrosis factor therapy in inflammatory bowel disease. *World J Gastroenterol*. 2009;15(17):2067-2073.

Kornbluth A, Sachar D. Ulcerative colitis practice guidelines in adults: American College of Gastroenterology, Practice Parameters Committee. *Am J Gastroenterol*. 2010;105(3): 501-523; quiz 524.

Lichtenstein G, Hanauer S, Sandborn WJ. Management of Crohn's disease in adults. *Am J Gastroenterol*. 2009;104(2): 465-483.

Complementary and Alternative Medicine

Joshua Korzenik, MD

The use of complementary and alternative medicine (CAM), as well as visits to alternative practitioners, continues to increase dramatically in the United States. This trend is particularly apparent in patients with chronic diseases, including individuals with IBD. Health care providers who care for patients with IBD should be aware of common CAM approaches and be knowledgeable about the information that exists regarding the safety and efficacy of these approaches so they can counsel their patients appropriately. This is particularly important because many patients do not volunteer information to their care providers that they are using alternative approaches. This chapter summarizes current trends in CAM use in IBD and provides a brief survey of commonly used therapies.

Dubinsky M, Friedman S.
Pocket Guide to IBD, Second Edition (pp 75-84).
© 2011 SLACK Incorporated

I. Conditions to Consider

- Chronic disease
- IBD
- Significant or severe adverse events related to a conventional medication

II. Questions to Ask

What is CAM?

- CAM is a broadly inclusive term referring to a wide variety of possible therapies outside the conventional biopsychosocial model of medicine. The therapies are as disparate as herbal therapy, prayer healing, dance therapy, visualization, and homeopathy.
- CAM therapies are being adopted increasingly by the mainstream in the United States; the borders between some CAM and conventional medications are becoming blurred.

How prevalent is CAM use?

- Two identical United States surveys conducted in 1991 and 1997 of the general population suggest an increase in CAM use in recent years.
  - According to the survey results, the use of at least one of 16 different CAM therapies in the previous year increased from 31% in 1991 to 41.6% in 1997.
  - Further, visits to an alternative medicine practitioner increased from 36.3% in 1991 to 46.3% in 1997.
  - The IBD population likely reflects this trend as well.

Do these figures differ from country to country?

- Surveys in different countries have estimated CAM use among individuals with IBD, as follows:
  - 31% (Cork, Ireland)
  - 47% (Berne, Switzerland)
  - 57% (Winnipeg, Canada)
  - 69% (Los Angeles, California)

Who among IBD patients uses CAM therapies or visits CAM practitioners?

- Those individuals with IBD most likely to use CAM therapies or visit a CAM practitioner cannot be easily profiled. Some studies of IBD patients have suggested the following:
  - Women are more likely than men to use CAM.
  - Older individuals tend to use prayer, diet, and exercise as therapeutic interventions more than younger individuals do.
  - Those with longer disease duration use CAM more than those with more recent disease onset.
  - Individuals who have significant or severe adverse events related to a conventional medication are more likely to use CAM.
  - Some studies have found that a higher educational level correlated with CAM use.

What motivates IBD patients to turn to CAM?

- The motivations for most IBD patients using these therapies are generally straightforward:
  - The desire to be more in control of their lives is a powerful factor in confronting a disease that has given them a sense of a lack of control.

- ○ Some describe that conventional medicine makes them passive participants in their own care.
- ○ Most individuals use CAM not as an exclusive choice or because of dissatisfaction with or rejection of conventional medication but as a genuinely complementary approach. They have turned to CAM out of a willingness or eagerness to do whatever seems reasonable to them to improve their condition and maintain their health.
- ○ Some describe a lack of effectiveness of conventional medicine as a strong motivating factor.
- • Most surveys do not find that disease activity correlates with the decision to use CAM.

Do IBD patients report their use of CAM to their physicians?

- • While a high percentage of individuals with IBD use CAM, many do not report this use to their physicians, even when asked.
- • Survey responses show that many individuals volunteer their use of CAM to their primary care physicians, but most do not tell their gastroenterologist without being prompted.

What types of CAM do IBD patients use? (Table 12-1)

- • Diet
- • Exercise
- • Mind healing (meditation, prayer, relaxation techniques, biofeedback)
- • Physical manipulation (acupuncture, massage, acupressure, chiropracty, massage)
- • Oral therapy (vitamins, herbals, probiotics, homeopathy)

Table 12-1. Partial List of Alternative Therapeutics in IBD

Oral Therapies

Vitamin supplements
Herbal supplements
   Aloe vera
   Cat's claw
   Soy-derived isoflavones
   Green tea
   Ginseng
   Slippery elm
   Boswellia serrata
   Calendula
   Chamomile
   Bach Flower Remedies

Alternative Medical Systems
Homeopathy Naturopathy Ayurveda Traditional Chinese medicine
Probiotics/Prebiotics
Nissle 1917 *Saccharomyces boulardii* VSL#3 PB8 Homeostatic Soil Organisms/Primal Defense
Diet
The Specific Carbohydrate Diet Low carbohydrate diet Rice water diet
Mind-Body Interventions
Relaxation techniques Prayer Meditation Distant healing

(continued)

Table 12-1. Partial List of Alternative
Therapeutics in IBD (continued)

Physical Manipulation/Exercise
Chiropracty/osteopathy
Feldenkrais
Aerobic exercise
Acupressure
Acupuncture
Reiki
Massage therapy
Therapeutic touch

Which therapies are most commonly used by IBD patients?

- Oral medications (including herbal remedies, which were used by 45% of respondents in one survey)
- Homeopathy (this is more popular in Europe than in North America, used by 52% in Switzerland, 16% in Canada)
- Chiropracty (41%)
- Massage therapy (23%)
- Prayer (17%)
- Relaxation techniques (17%)

What are the most popular herbal supplements among IBD patients?

- Aloe vera, an oral medication, is frequently used, with some evidence suggesting that it helps to improve healing. A placebo-controlled trial suggested a benefit in ulcerative colitis (UC).

- *Boswellia serrata,* or Indian frankincense, is also popular. It has been studied in controlled trials in both Crohn's disease and collagenous colitis.
- Curcumin has been studied for maintenance of remission in UC.
- Other herbal supplements that are often used include:
  - Cat's claw (*Uncaria tomentosa*)
  - Slippery elm
  - Ginseng
  - Green tea
  - Soy-derived isoflavones
- Although some animal data support the theoretical use of some of these compounds, human studies have not been performed.
- An attraction of these medications is that they are "natural" and therefore presumed to be benign or virtually free of side effects. Unfortunately, however, these medications (herbals or others) do have potentially mild and serious side effects. *The Physicians' Desk Reference for Herbal Medicines* is a useful reference.

What are some of the diets that IBD patients follow?

- The Specific Carbohydrate Diet (Gottschall diet)
- Low carbohydrate diets
- Rice water diets
- These approaches have not been adequately studied to cite reliable supporting data outside of anecdotal reports.

Has acupuncture been studied as a treatment for IBD?

- Acupuncture, best evaluated for its analgesic effect, has been studied for the treatment of UC and Crohn's disease in China, where these diseases appear to be increasing.

What are probiotics and prebiotics?

- Probiotics are live organisms that confer a health benefit. Prebiotics are mostly complex carbohydrates that selectively stimulate the growth or activity of potentially beneficial bacteria.
- Probiotics and prebiotics are making a transition from being on the edge of CAM to part of mainstream medicine, particularly with regard to gastrointestinal diseases.
- The particular species and dose, as with any medicine, are critical.
  - Probiotics (usually strains of *Bifidobacterium* or *Lactobacillus*) sold as supplements in health food stores usually contain 10^9 to 10^{10} (1 to 10 billion) organisms per dose. Although this is seemingly a large amount, 1 g of stool contains between 10^{11} to 10^{12} (100 billion to 1 trillion) bacteria.

Does stress play a role in IBD?

- Although stress is considered by many patients to play a central role in provoking flares of IBD, the data to support this contention have been inconsistent. Regardless of whether the stress is causative in IBD, stress reduction through mind-body techniques and other approaches may have a benefit.

III. Conclusion

Many people are drawn to the use of CAM therapies by the perception that these approaches hold the promise of benefit without adverse effects and also because they have experienced side effects with conventional medications or are otherwise unsatisfied with their response to conventional therapy. As with conventional medications, however, these approaches should not be used cavalierly. With any medication, doses, duration of treatment, preparations, and potential interactions are all critical factors that need to be evaluated and understood, although there are few well-conducted studies to guide the use of alternative compounds. Unfortunately, most CAM approaches rely primarily on anecdotal reports spread through word of mouth or Internet chat boards. Reliance on anecdotal evidence causes potentially very useful compounds such as probiotics to be mixed in with reports of benefits promoting things as unlikely as gummy bears and coconut cookies as treatments for IBD; however, some of these approaches likely are of benefit. If CAM approaches are useful to patients with IBD, even if based on a very different theoretical framework of disease and health, they should be able to be studied to determine whether they are useful, to help guide their use by people with IBD.

Suggested Readings

García-Vega E, Fernandez-Rodriguez C. A stress management programme for Crohn's disease. *Behav Res Ther.* 2004;42(4):367-383.

Gerhardt H, Seifert F, Buvari P, Vogelsang H. Therapy of active Crohn disease with *Boswellia serrata* extract H 15 [in German]. *Z Gastroenterol.* 2001;39(1):11-17.

Gionchetti P, Rizzello F, Venturi A, et al. Oral bacteriotherapy as maintenance treatment in patients with chronic pouchitis: a double-blind, placebo-controlled trial. *Gastroenterology.* 2000;119(2):305-309.

Hanai H, Iida T, Takeuchi K, et al. Curcumin maintenance therapy for ulcerative colitis: randomized, multicenter, double-blind, placebo-controlled trial. *Clin Gastroenterol Hepatol.* 2006;4(12):1502-1506.

Hilsden RJ, Verhoef MJ, Best A, Pocobelli G. Complementary and alternative medicine use by Canadian patients with inflammatory bowel disease: results from a national survey. *Am J Gastroenterol.* 2003;98(7):1563-1568.

Joos S, Wildau N, Kohnen R, et al. Acupuncture and moxibustion in the treatment of ulcerative colitis: a randomized controlled study. *Scand J Gastroenterol.* 2006;41(9):1056-1063.

Kessler RC, Davis RB, Foster DF, et al. Long-term trends in the use of complementary and alternative medical therapies in the United States. *Ann Intern Med.* 2001;135(4):262-268.

Langhorst J, Mueller T, Luedtke R, et al. Effects of a comprehensive lifestyle modification program on quality-of-life in patients with ulcerative colitis: a twelve-month follow-up. *Scand J Gastroenterol.* 2007;42(6):734-745.

Langmead L, Feakins RM, Goldthorpe S, et al. Randomized, double-blind, placebo-controlled trial of oral aloe vera gel for active ulcerative colitis. *Aliment Pharmacol Ther.* 2004;19(7): 739-747.

Madisch A, Miehlke S, Eichele O, et al. *Boswellia serrata* extract for the treatment of collagenous colitis: a double-blind, randomized, placebo-controlled, multicenter trial. *Int J Colorectal Dis.* 2007;22(12):1445-1451.

Quattropani C, Ausfeld B, Straumann A, Heer P, Seibold F. Complementary alternative medicine in patients with inflammatory bowel disease: use and attitudes. *Scand J Gastroenterol.* 2003;38(3):277-282.

Rawsthorne P, Shanahan F, Cronin NC, et al. An international survey of the use and attitudes regarding alternative medicine by patients with inflammatory bowel disease. *Am J Gastroenterol.* 1999;94(5):1298-1303.

Rembacken BJ, Snelling AM, Hawkey PM, Chalmers DM, Axon AT. Non-pathogenic *Escherichia coli* versus mesalazine for the treatment of ulcerative colitis: a randomised trial. *Lancet.* 1999;354(9179):635-639.

SECTION IV

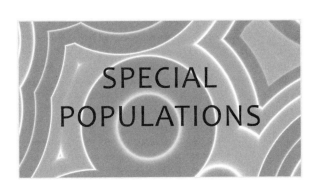

SPECIAL POPULATIONS

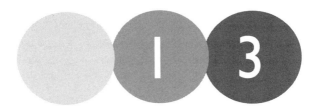

The Postoperative Patient

Judy F. Collins, MD

The patient with IBD who has just had surgery may have problems with wound pain, bowel recovery, or discomfort related to drains. When these patients call, it is helpful to know what type of surgery they have had, when it was done, and what their symptoms are. If the surgery involved any type of bowel resection, then the first things to consider are wound dehiscence, infection, abscess formation, anastomotic leak, ischemia of the anastomosis, and small bowel obstruction. Symptomatic disease recurrence tends to occur months after resection, but if the patient has a retained rectum or retained involved bowel, some of his or her symptoms may indeed be secondary to active IBD immediately postoperatively. Any patient who has had recent surgery and calls with nausea, vomiting, abdominal distention, and decreased output should be seen immediately to evaluate for obstruction or loss of bowel continuity. An in-person assessment is always helpful, and a discussion with the patient's surgeon is

Dubinsky M, Friedman S.
Pocket Guide to IBD, Second Edition (pp 87-94).
© 2011 SLACK Incorporated

usually prudent if the symptoms occur within the first 30 days after surgery.

Another issue that will come up after surgery concerns initiation or restarting of medical treatment. In general, medical treatment should be started within 3 to 4 weeks following surgery if the patient has had more than 2 surgeries already or has perforating or significant stricturing disease.

A repeat colonoscopy is recommended 6 months postoperatively to assess for recurrence or progression of disease. This may give a 3- to 6-month advance notice of recurrence. In cases where the disease is not accessible by colonoscopy, a small bowel imaging study can be considered within 6 to 12 months after surgery.

I. CONDITIONS TO CONSIDER

- Wound dehiscence/infection
- Abscess formation
- Anastomotic leak
- Ischemia of anastomosis
- Small bowel obstruction
- Acute narcotic withdrawal
- *Clostridium difficile*
- Recurrent disease

II. QUESTIONS TO ASK

What are the patient's current symptoms?

- Fever, nausea/vomiting, increased fecal/stoma/fistula output, decreased output, bleeding from rectum or stoma, and pain (characterize location, duration, pattern). May suggest an anastomotic leak, wound infection, or abscess formation. Immediate evaluation is recommended.

- It is sometimes possible to tell, during the initial telephone conversation, whether the patient's complaint is a medical or surgical issue, and the patient can be referred to the surgeon when appropriate. Any complaints about the surgical wound or stoma should be referred back to the surgeon.

When did the surgery take place?

- The differential changes when the surgery was 1 week ago versus 2 months ago.

What type of surgery was performed, and what is the current anatomy?

- *Small bowel resection with primary anastomosis.* Consider leak, ischemia, or stricture.
- *Small bowel resection with diverting ileostomy.* Consider obstruction or leak/ischemia of rectal stump.
- *Colonic resection with primary anastomosis.* Consider anastomotic leak/ischemia.
- *Colonic resection with small bowel ileostomy.* Consider ischemia of distal ileum and abdominal wall problems; assess for retraction of the stoma.
- *Drainage of abscess.* Consider reaccumulation of abscess or the drain not in position.
- *Stage 1 or 2 surgery with ileal pouch anal anastomosis.* Consider leak/ischemia. (For ulcerative colitis, an ileal pouch anal anastomosis will be performed in stages, and a retained rectum can bleed.)
- Intra-abdominal abscess is always a consideration.

- Postoperative urinary tract infections, pneumonias, and pulmonary embolus should also be considered.

What medications is the patient taking?

- Patients taking a significant amount of narcotics can develop constipation, ileus, and small bowel obstruction. Acute withdrawal from narcotics can cause rebound pain or withdrawal-type symptoms.
- A patient with Crohn's disease who has not restarted maintenance medications may have an early recurrence if some of the disease has not been resected.
- Nonsteroidal medications may lead to anastomotic ulcers and bleeding, independent of any IBD.

What is the patient's current diet?

- Premature advancement of diet or nonadherence to a low-residue diet in the early postoperative period can lead to small bowel obstruction or diarrhea.

III. TESTS AND ASSESSMENTS TO ORDER

- *Physical examination.* A patient complaining of an infected wound, fever, obstructive symptoms, or abdominal pain or distension should be promptly evaluated. Check the patient's temperature, blood pressure, and pulse. Assess pain level. Conduct an abdominal examination. Check the appearance of the wound/stoma. Look for rectal swelling, redness, whether setons are present, and the type of discharge.

- Laboratory tests
  - Complete blood cell count with differential
  - Electrolyte panel
  - Amylase and lipase
  - Consider wound and blood cultures
  - Consider stool culture for *C difficile* toxin
  - Consider urine culture and sensitivity
- X-rays
  - Chest x-ray for infiltrates if the patient had a Foley catheter and/or limited activity, poor nutritional status, or was on steroids; will also assess for free air
  - Supine and upright abdominal films to rule out small bowel obstruction
  - Computed tomography scan of the abdomen and pelvis to rule out abscess formation, free fluid, and pancreatitis
- Endoscopy
  - Rarely needed in the early postoperative period, as there will be edema secondary to the surgery itself and not necessarily indicative of active disease
  - Helpful weeks to months postoperatively to rule out recurrent disease or ulcerations from other causes; can perform colonoscopy via rectum, colostomy, or ileostomy if appropriate; highly recommended 6 months postoperatively to look for endoscopic disease recurrence prior to onset of symptoms. Recurrence can be seen as early as 4 weeks postoperatively.

IV. Postoperative Medical Treatment

- Medical treatment of aggressive disease is probably indicated and is recommended if the patient has had more than 2 surgeries or has stricturing/perforating disease. At a minimum, the patient should have an endoscopy at 6 months to look for recurrence of disease. If more than aphthous ulcers or scattered discrete ulcers is found, consider medical prophylaxis/treatment.
- Metronidazole 20 mg/kg orally or ornidazole 500mg orally twice daily, started within 1 to 3 weeks postoperatively may diminish early endoscopic recurrence for up to 12 months.
- Mesalamine administered in doses greater than 4 g/day postoperatively for the prevention of recurrent ileocolonic disease may have shown some benefit in 2 studies; most studies have used doses less than 4.8 g/day. However, most evidence-based studies do not support the use of mesalamine for postoperative prophylaxis.
- Administration of azathioprine 2.5 mg/kg or 6-mercaptopurine (6-MP) 1.5 mg/kg (one study used 6-MP 50-mg flat dose) has shown a decrease in recurrence of ileocolonic disease at 12 months when started within 4 weeks after surgery.
- Administration of tumor necrosis factor-alpha inhibitors may decrease recurrence of disease when given within 4 to 8 weeks after surgery.

Suggested Readings

Ferrante M, D'Hoore A, Vermeire S, et al. Corticosteroids but not infliximab increase short-term postoperative infectious complications in patients with ulcerative colitis. *Inflamm Bowel Dis.* 2009; 15(7):1062-1070.

Gorfine SR, Fichera A, Harris MT, Bauer JJ. Long-term results of salvage surgery for septic complications after restorative proctocolectomy: does fecal diversion improve outcome? *Dis Colon Rectum.* 2003;46(10):1339-1344.

Issa M, Ananthakrishnayan AN, Binion DG. Clostridium difficile and inflammatory bowel disease. *Inflamm Bowel Dis.* 2008;14(10):1432-1442.

Lundeen SJ, Otterson MF, Binion DG, Carman ET, Peppard WJ. Clostridium difficile enteritis: an early postoperative complication in inflammatory bowel disease patients after colectomy. *J Gastrointest Surg.* 2007;11(2):138-142.

Mahadevan U, Loftus EV, Tremaine WJ, et al. Azathioprine or 6-mercaptopurine before colectomy for ulcerative colitis is not associated with increased postoperative complications. *Inflamm Bowel Dis.* 2002;8(5):311-316.

Ng SC, Kamm MA. Management of postoperative Crohn's disease. *Am J Gastroenterol.* 2008;103(4):1029-1035.

Peyrin-Biroulet L, Dettenre P, Ardizzone S, et al. Azathioprine and 6-mercaptopurine for the prevention of postoperative recurrence in Crohn's disease: a meta-analysis. *Am J Gastroenterol.* 2009;104(8):2089-2096.

Regueiro, M. Management and prevention of postoperative Crohn's disease. *Inflamm Bowel Dis.* 2009;15(10):1583-1590.

Regueiro M, Schraut W, Baidoo L, et al. Infliximab prevents Crohn's disease recurrence after ileal resection. *Gastroenterology.* 2009;136(2):144-450.

Rutgeerts P, Van Assche G, Vermeire S, et al. Ornidazole for prophylaxis of postoperative Crohn's disease recurrence: a randomized, double-blind, placebo controlled trial of ornidazole. *Gastroenterology.* 2005;128(4):856-861.

Schwartz M, Regueiro M. Prevention and treatment of postoperative Crohn's disease recurrence: an update for a new decade. *Curr Gastroenterol Rep.* 2010;126(5):246e-248e.

Selvasekar CR, Cima RR, Larson DW, et al. Effect of infliximab on short-term complications in patients undergoing operation for chronic ulcerative colitis. *J Am Coll Surg.* 2007;204(5):956-962.

Subramanian V, Pollok RC, Kang JY, Kumar D. Systematic review of postoperative complications in patients with inflammatory bowel disease treated with immunomodulators. *Brit J Surg.* 2006;93(7):793-799.

Subramanian V, Saxena S, Kang JY, Pollok RC. Preoperative steroid use and risk of postoperative complications in patients with inflammatory bowel disease undergoing abdominal surgery. *Am J Gastroenterol.* 2008;103(9):2373-2381.

Velayos FS, Sandborn WJ. Use of azathioprine and 6-mercaptopurine in postoperative Crohn's disease: changing natural history or just along for the ride? *Am J Gastroenterol.* 2009; 104(8):2097-2099.

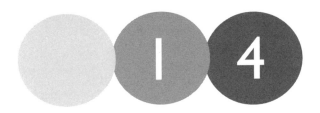

The Patient
With a Pouch

Bo Shen, MD

A pouch, or ileal pouch, is created during bowel reconstruction surgery following total proctocolectomy for patients with ulcerative colitis (UC) or familial adenomatous polyposis. Approximately one-third of patients with UC eventually require colectomy for medically refractory disease or dysplasia. Restorative proctocolectomy with ileal pouch–anal anastomosis (IPAA) has become the surgical procedure of choice for patients with colectomy. This procedure significantly reduces the patient's risk for dysplasia or cancer and improves the patient's health-related quality of life. Typically, patients with healthy pouches have 4 to 7 soft bowel movements a day without incontinence, cramps, or nocturnal symptoms. However, inflammatory and noninflammatory complications of the pouch often occur. If a patient has increased bowel frequency, watery stool, abdominal cramps, bloating, pelvic discomfort, and/or incontinence, he or she may have inflammatory or functional complications of the pouch. The

Dubinsky M, Friedman S.
Pocket Guide to IBD, Second Edition (pp 95-100).
© 2011 SLACK Incorporated

most common inflammatory complications are pouchitis, cuffitis, and Crohn's disease (CD) of the pouch.

I. Conditions to Consider

- Pouchitis
- Cuffitis
- CD of the pouch
- Irritable pouch syndrome
- Infectious diarrhea from bacterial or viral pathogens, particularly *Clostridium difficile*–associated pouchitis
- Concurrent celiac disease
- Nonsteroidal anti-inflammatory drug (NSAID)–induced pouchopathy

II. Questions to Ask

What are the patient's predominant symptoms?

- *Increased bowel frequency, change in stool consistency, urgency, seepage, nocturnal symptoms, and abdominal cramps*. These symptoms are not specific for any of the inflammatory or functional disorders of the ileal pouch.
- *Blood in the stool*. This is a typical presentation in patients with cuffitis; it seldom occurs in patients with pouchitis.
- *Fever, general malaise, weight loss, and dehydration*. These symptoms are not a common presentation in patients with conventional pouchitis, which is believed to be triggered by an alteration in commensal bacteria of the pouch. For patients with these symptoms, infectious

pathogens, such as *C difficile*, cytomegalovirus, and *Campylobacter* species, should be excluded.

Are there any associated symptoms?

- Nausea, vomiting, bloating, early satiety, and dyschezia may indicate partial small bowel obstruction resulting from surgical adhesions, small bowel or anastomotic strictures, or anismus.
- Persistent diarrhea and weight loss despite aggressive antibiotic therapy may indicate CD of the pouch or celiac disease.

Are there other behaviors that may be contributing to the problem?

- Use of broad-spectrum antibiotics, particularly those for respiratory infection, can trigger pouchitis.
- Long-term use of ciprofloxacin or metronidazole may be associated with an increased risk for *C difficile* infection of the pouch. Therefore, metronidazole is not used as first-line therapy for *C difficile*–associated pouchitis.
- NSAID use can trigger or exacerbate symptoms of pouchitis.
- A diet with a high content of simple sugar may be associated with symptoms of bloating and diarrhea.
- Smoking has been reported to be associated with an increased risk for CD of the pouch.
- Some female patients may notice a pattern of more active symptoms of the pouch related to their menstrual cycle.

What are current therapies for inflammatory and functional pouch disorder?

- There are no Food and Drug Administration–approved agents for pouch disorders. All clinically used agents are off-label applications.
- Antibiotic therapy is the main treatment modality for pouchitis. Commonly used agents include ciprofloxacin, metronidazole, rifaximin, and tinidazole. For the majority of patients with pouchitis, a 2-week course of a single antibiotic agent is sufficient. However, some patients may require long-term maintenance therapy with antibiotics. Alternatively, these patients may benefit from probiotic therapy to keep the disease in remission. A subset of patients may develop antibiotic resistance. For these patients, 5-aminosalicylate agents (ASAs), topically active corticosteroids (such as budesonide), immunomodulators, and even biologic agents may be tried.
- Cuffitis is typically treated with topical 5-ASAs or topical corticosteroids.
- For CD of the pouch, particularly fibrostenotic and fistulizing phenotypes, 5-ASAs, corticosteroids, immunomodulators, and biologic agents have been used. A combined medical, endoscopic, and surgical therapy is often needed for fibrostenotic and fistulizing CD of the pouch.
- For irritable pouch syndrome, the most common form of functional disorder in patients with IPAA, treatment regimens include antispasmodics, tricyclic antidepressants, and opium tincture.

III. TESTS AND ASSESSMENTS TO ORDER

- Flexible pouchoscopy is the most accurate modality for the diagnosis and differential diagnosis of ileal pouch disorder.
- Biopsies should be taken from the neo-terminal ileum, pouch body, and anal transitional zone. The main purposes for histologic evaluation are to identify granulomas (for the diagnosis of CD), viral inclusion bodies (for cytomegalovirus infection), ischemia, prolapse, and dysplasia.
- Laboratory studies
  - Stool studies should be obtained for *C difficile* toxin A and B and bacterial culture, particularly in patients with persistent or systemic symptoms and long-term use of antibiotics or immunosuppressive agents.
  - Periodic monitoring with a complete blood cell count and liver function tests is advocated. Approximately 25% of patients with IPAA have some degree of anemia, approximately 10% have transient or persistent elevation of liver enzymes, and approximately 5% have concurrent primary sclerosing cholangitis.
- Imaging studies
  - Computed tomography (CT), CT enterography, magnetic resonance imaging of the pelvis, and water-soluble contrast enemas are commonly used diagnostic modalities in evaluation of structural abnormalities of the pouch, such as stricture, fistula, pouch sinus, pouch leak, and pelvic abscess.

SUGGESTED READINGS

Shen B, Fazio VW, Remzi FH, et al. Comprehensive evaluation of inflammatory and non-inflammatory sequelae of ileal pouch-anal anastomosis. *Am J Gastroenterol.* 2005;100(1): 93-101.

Shen B, Remzi FH, Lavery IC, Lashner BA, Fazio VW. A proposed classification of ileal pouch disorders and associated complications after restorative proctocolectomy. *Clin Gastroenterol Hepatol.* 2008;6(2):145-158.

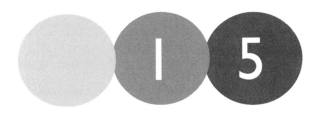

The Patient
With an Ostomy

Nimisha K. Parekh, MD

Patients with ulcerative colitis undergoing an ileal pouch–anal anastomosis will have a temporary ostomy, and certain patients with Crohn's disease may undergo a temporary or permanent ileostomy or colostomy. Between 6% and 66% of these patients will have stoma-related issues. Living with a stoma can be difficult for a patient due to fear and change in body image, as well as complications. Routine follow up to check the function of the stoma, the integrity of the pouching system, and the patient's physical and emotional well-being is essential for the prevention of, and early interventions for, ostomy complications. The care of a patient with an ostomy is best coordinated with a multidisciplinary team including an ostomy/wound nurse, an enterostomal therapist, the surgeon, and the gastroenterologist.

Dubinsky M, Friedman S.
Pocket Guide to IBD, Second Edition (pp 101-106).
© 2011 SLACK Incorporated

I. Conditions to Consider

- Allergic or chemical reaction
- Stomal complications (hernia, prolapse, necrosis, protrusion)
- Rashes (folliculitis, *Candida* infection, pyoderma gangrenosum)
- Bowel obstruction
- Recurrent disease
- High output from ostomy/dehydration

II. Questions to Ask

What type of ostomy is in place?

- *Ileostomy* is a stoma created after removal of the colon to connect the ileum to an external pouching system. The stoma is usually in the right lower quadrant. The fecal matter is often semiliquid.
- *Continent ileostomy*, or Koch pouch, is made with a loop of ileum that is brought up to the skin and closed off by a nipple valve. The valve allows access for emptying and eliminates the need for an external pouching system. The Koch pouch is rarely used today.
- *Colostomy* is a loop of colon that is brought up to the skin and attached to a pouching system. It can be created anywhere in the colon.
- *Double-barrel colostomy* has 2 stomas: one stoma is present to drain the fecal matter to an external pouching system, and the second is a mucous fistula that drains mucus and is covered with a gauze dressing.

How does the stoma appear?

- The stoma should appear beefy red. If the stoma appears brown, purple, or black, the surgeon should be notified immediately for concerns of ischemia.
- The stoma should protrude only slightly. A retracted stoma has sunk below skin level. If this occurs, a special type of pouching system needs to be used. A prolapsed stoma can protrude several inches into the pouching system. If this occurs, the mucosa can become edematous and deep red in color.

How does the skin around the stoma appear?

- The skin around the stoma should be assessed. If the skin is raw, moist, or irritated, there is most likely leakage and fecal irritation of the skin or an allergic reaction. The patient may complain of itching and burning as well. The pouching system needs to be evaluated, and stoma powders or paste may need to be used.
- Pustules, papules, or severe redness noted around the stoma could indicate peristomal candidiasis or folliculitis. If the pustules open and progress to full ulcers with irregular edges, the presentation is one of peristomal pyoderma gangrenosum.
- Rare skin disorders of the peristomal skin include herpes, pemphigus, and psoriasis.

What is the output from stoma?

- The output can vary but typically ranges from 500 to 1500 mL in a 24-hour period. Greater outputs can lead to dehydration. Ileostomy patients are at risk for dehydration and should be educated to monitor for signs of dehydration, including dry skin, thirst, cramps, rapid heart rate, and confusion. Patients should see their physician immediately for these issues.

- If there is no liquid or gas output, the patient should be evaluated for a bowel obstruction.
- If the patient complains of constipation, explosive gas, or pain at the time of stoma emptying, evaluate for stenosis.
- If the patient has significant output and fevers, consider infectious etiologies.

What is the patient's current medical regimen?

- Nonsteroidal anti-inflammatory use is associated with a flare in IBD.
- Topical medications can lead to hypersensitivity reactions.
- Many complementary and alternative medicines have unknown effects and toxicities.
- Time-released medications may not release effectively and empty into the pouch, rendering them essentially ineffective.

Is there bleeding?

- Blood mixed with fecal output suggests active disease.
- Clots may indicate active bleeding; the presence of clots requires immediate attention and evaluation.
- Bleeding in the surrounding skin suggests skin irritation or rash.
- A purple hue around the stoma with intermittent bleeding or profuse bleeding into the pouch can

indicate peristomal varices. This condition is seen in patients who have portal hypertension or cirrhosis of the liver.

How long has the bleeding been going on?

- Patients often wait before calling the office. If the bleeding has been persistent, the patient should be educated to seek immediate medical attention.

III. TESTS AND ASSESSMENTS TO ORDER

- *Physical examination.* Assess the stoma color, opening, and protrusion, the peristomal skin, and the pouching system. Check the patient's skin turgor, heart rate, blood pressure, and overall appearance.
- Laboratory studies
  - Complete blood cell count to assess chronicity and severity of bleeding
  - Basic metabolic panel and electrolyte panel to help with assessment and treatment of dehydration
  - C-reactive protein and erythrocyte sedimentation rate to evaluate for inflammation
- Endoscopic evaluation through the stoma allows for direct visualization and the ability to obtain biopsies to evaluate for active disease and infection. If bleeding is profuse, the patient may also need an upper endoscopy.

IV. OTHER PEARLS FOR PATIENTS WITH AN OSTOMY

- Activities
  - Patients can participate in a wide range of activities, including running, swimming, horseback riding, and many more, as they did prior to ostomy placement. Heavy weightlifting should be discussed with the physician. Bathing and showering can be done with or without the pouching system. Clothing does not pose a problem; special underwear and covers are made for the pouch systems.
  - Patients are often hesitant to discuss concerns about sexual activity with an ostomy. Concerns range from anxiety to questions about reproductive issues and actual process. The patient and partner should discuss these issues with the enterostomal nurse and, if needed, an enterostomal therapist.
- Traveling tips for a patient with an ostomy
  - The best advice for the patient is to be prepared. The patient should pack extra supplies, and if traveling to areas with different climates, he or she should ask the enterostomal therapist or physician about the local food and water. Water that is safe for drinking is usually okay for irrigation.

SUGGESTED READING

Colwell J. Stomal and peristomal skin complications. In: Colwell J, Goldberg M, Carmel J, eds. *Fecal and Urinary Diversions: Management Principles*. St. Louis, MO: Mosby; 2004:308-325.

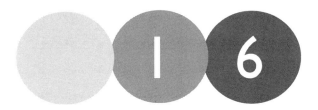

The Pediatric Patient

Marla Dubinsky, MD

Children account for approximately 25% of all IBD cases. The median age at diagnosis is 11 years. Crohn's disease (CD) is primarily seen in children of school age, outnumbering ulcerative colitis (UC) by approximately 3 to 1, but in children of preschool age, UC or IBD unspecified (IBDU) is as frequent as CD. Although the clinical manifestations of IBD among children or adults may be very similar, key features of pediatric-onset disease distinguish this population as unique.

I. CONDITIONS TO CONSIDER

- Growth failure
- Pubertal delay
- Proximal small bowel involvement
- Medication adherence
- Complex communication matrix
- Fear of procedures
- Depression and anxiety
- School absenteeism

Dubinsky M, Friedman S.
Pocket Guide to IBD, Second Edition (pp 107-114).
© 2011 SLACK Incorporated

- Family history
- Colon cancer risk
- Lack of indicated therapies

II. Questions to Ask

Does the child have growth failure?

- At least one-third of children with CD yet only one-tenth of children with UC present with growth failure. The presence of growth failure must increase the suspicion for CD involving the small bowel even in the face of what is considered an established diagnosis of UC.
- Growth failure can occur prior to the onset of any gastrointestinal symptoms.
- The most common cause of growth failure is malnutrition, which is primarily a result of inadequate caloric intake. Other causes of malnutrition include increased intestinal losses, malabsorption, and increased energy requirements.
- Weight loss typically precedes linear growth failure.
- Pubertal delay is another manifestation of malnutrition and often accompanies linear growth delay.
- Active disease can contribute to ongoing growth failure.
- Corticosteroids can have a significant effect on growth velocity, and steroid dependency remains an unacceptable therapeutic end point for pediatric patients.
- Genetic and endocrine factors can certainly impact growth and must be considered in the differential diagnosis of growth failure.

Are children adhering to their medications?

- Illness-related, patient-related, family-related, and physician-related factors influence treatment adherence.
- The stage and course of the illness will impact treatment adherence.
- The psychological state of mind of the child will impact the adherence to treatment, with positive self-esteem being an important predictor of adherence.
- The quality of family functioning will affect the adherence to therapies, and family disruption must be monitored.
- The importance of articulating a clear treatment plan cannot be underscored enough when talking about ways to maximize patient and family adherence.
- Physicians need to appreciate that socioeconomic class and ethnicity may influence beliefs and impact adherence to medical management.
- Peer support groups can enhance adherence through the exchange of medical information.
- Teens generally acquire negotiation tools that differ from those for the younger age group, and maintaining autonomy is important for adherence in teenagers.
- Decreasing pill count and simplifying the timing of pill taking can increase medication compliance.

What is the psychosocial impact of IBD on the child?

- Maximizing the quality of life is an important outcome in the treatment of IBD patients.

- Children with IBD strive to "fit in" and to not be different from their peers.
- It is uncommon for children with IBD to disclose their illness to children unaffected by IBD or other chronic diseases.
- School absenteeism secondary to illness and hospitalizations can impact school performance and peer relationships.
- The esthetic and emotional side effects of certain medications, corticosteroids in particular, can significantly affect the psychosocial functioning of children.
- Depression and anxiety are not uncommon in children with IBD.
- Support groups and national camp programs may play a very important role in helping children and their families cope with disease and improve psychosocial functioning.

Is the natural history of IBD in children different from that in adults?

- Disease onset before the age of 15 and disease duration are known risk factors for the development of colon cancer in UC.
- Chemopreventive measures with 5-aminosalicylate therapies and folic acid should be considered early in the course of disease.
- Screening colonoscopy needs to be used in children after 8 years of age for extensive colitis and after 10 years of age for left-sided colitis.
- The screening regimen for children with primary sclerosing cholangitis and colitis should start at the time of diagnosis.
- CD onset before the age of 20 has been shown to be associated with a more aggressive disease course with patients undergoing more surgeries due to medically refractory disease.

- Immunomodulators and biologics may be considered early in children presenting with extensive disease, steroid dependency, and growth failure.

Are the therapies used in children different from those used in adults?

- The therapeutic approach for children is essentially the same as for adults with IBD.
- Both induction and maintenance therapies are used in children.
- The only therapies currently approved for use in children with IBD are corticosteroids, sulfasalazine, and infliximab.
- Mesalamine-based therapies remain first-line therapies in patients with mild to moderate IBD with colonic involvement.
- Nutritional supplementation is an important part of the treatment of a child, especially in the face of growth failure.
- Corticosteroids, although frequently used, can have a significant impact on growth, and thus only short-term courses are used. There is no role for low-dose corticosteroids for the maintenance of disease remission.
- Immunomodulators, such as 6-mercaptopurine/azathioprine and methotrexate, are very effective therapies used for the maintenance of steroid-free remission.
- Infliximab is frequently used in children, and its efficacy appears superior to that seen in adults (88% response rate). The safety profile parallels that for adults, with most patients tolerating this therapy.

- Infectious complications need to be monitored in all patients taking immunosuppressants, including corticosteroids.
- All immunosuppressed patients should receive an annual flu shot.
- Children on immunomodulators should not receive live vaccines.
- The surgical approaches to children with both CD and UC are similar to those in adults.

III. TESTS AND ASSESSMENTS TO ORDER

In addition to the common endoscopic, radiologic, and laboratory tests that are ordered for all IBD patients, certain tests may help to optimize the management of pediatric patients with IBD.

- Calorie count and nutritional consult can help to ensure adequate caloric intake and prevent growth failure.
- Albumin, prealbumin, an iron panel, and vitamin D levels can provide a very good baseline assessment of nutritional status and degree of malabsorption.
- A bone age study in a child who presents with growth failure can provide information on catch-up growth potential when compared to chronological age.
- A bone density scan may not be very accurate in children if not compared to the appropriate age- and sex-matched population. A quantitative computed tomography (CT) scan may be more accurate, as it describes a three-dimensional image and examines bone volume.
- Video capsule endoscopy is a noninvasive method to assess small bowel inflammation.

- CT scans should be used only when necessary in children given the cumulative radiation exposure risk over their lifetime. Magnetic resonance imaging is emerging as the radiologic evaluation of choice in pediatrics.
- Serologic immune markers for IBD (ie, anti-*Saccharomyces cerevisiae* antibodies, antineutrophil antibodies, and anti-outer membrane porin C) may be helpful in differentiating CD from UC in patients presenting with IBDU and for predicting the natural history of the disease.
- Fecal calprotectin is a noninvasive test that may be helpful in predicting response to treatment and relapse in patients with IBD.
- A psychosocial evaluation for the patient and his or her family can be an important part of the overall management of patients with IBD.

Suggested Readings

Dubinsky MC, Kugathasan S, Mei L, et al. Increased immune reactivity predicts aggressive complicating Crohn's disease in children. *Clin Gastroenterol Hepatol.* 2008;6(10):1105-1111.

Hyams J, Crandall W, Kugathasan S, et al. Induction and maintenance infliximab therapy for the treatment of moderate-to-severe Crohn's disease in children. *Gastroenterology.* 2007;132(3):863–873; quiz 1165-1166.

Imielinski M, Baldassano RN, Griffiths A, et al. Common variants at five new loci associated with early-onset inflammatory bowel disease. *Nat Genet.* 2009;41(12):1335-1340.

Thayu M, Denson LA, Shults J, et al. Determinants of changes in linear growth and body composition in incident pediatric Crohn's disease. *Gastroenterology.* 2010;139(2):430-438.

Vasseur F, Gower-Rousseau C, Vernier-Massouille G, et al. Nutritional status and growth in pediatric Crohn's disease: a population-based study. *Am J Gastroenterol.* 2010;105(8):1893-1900.

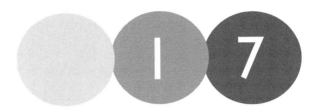

The Pregnant Patient

Uma Mahadevan, MD

The highest age-adjusted incidence rates of IBD overlap the peak reproductive years. New medications are allowing patients to be healthier and disease free for longer intervals, which may prompt a desire for conception. A pregnant IBD patient should be carefully monitored by both her gastroenterologist and her obstetrician for signs of active disease and fetal complications.

I. CONDITIONS TO CONSIDER

- Fertility
  - Women with ulcerative colitis (UC) and Crohn's disease (CD) have similar rates of fertility compared to the general population.
  - Surgical intervention in the pelvis, such as a proctocolectomy with ileoanal pouch, can decrease fertility.

Dubinsky M, Friedman S.
Pocket Guide to IBD, Second Edition (pp 115-124).
© 2011 SLACK Incorporated

- Disease activity
  - The chances of having a disease flare during pregnancy are the same as in the nonpregnant woman—33% per year.
  - Women should be in remission prior to contemplating conception.
  - Disease activity during pregnancy may increase the risk of preterm birth and spontaneous abortion.
  - Even if disease activity is in remission, women with IBD have higher rates of adverse pregnancy outcomes than the general population.
- Pregnancy outcome
  - In general, women with IBD have healthy pregnancies and healthy infants.
  - Women with IBD do have higher rates of spontaneous abortion, premature birth, low birth weight, and complications of labor and delivery.
  - Women with IBD should be monitored as high-risk obstetric patients.
- Fetal outcome
  - The majority of infants are normal and healthy.
  - There is an increased risk of low-birth-weight and preterm infants.
  - Congenital malformations do not appear to be higher, although the data are mixed.

II. QUESTIONS TO ASK

What medications are safe for the pregnant IBD patient to use? (Table 17-1)

Table 17-1. Medications Used in the Treatment of IBD: Recommendations for Pregnancy and Breastfeeding

Drug	Food and Drug Administration Category	Recommendations for Pregnancy	Breastfeeding
Adalimumab	B	Limited human data, low risk* Likely crosses placenta	Minimal transfer Probably compatible
Alendronate	C	Limited human data, long half-life Animal data suggest risk	No human data Probably compatible
Azathioprine/ 6-mercaptopurine	D	Data in IBD and transplant literature suggest some risk, but low	Limited transfer Likely compatible
Balsalazide	B	Low risk	No human data Potential diarrhea

(continued)

Table 17-1. Medications Used in the Treatment of IBD:
Recommendations for Pregnancy and Breastfeeding (continued)

Drug	Food and Drug Administration Category	Recommendations for Pregnancy	Breastfeeding
Budesonide	C	Data with inhaled drug, low risk Limited human data for oral drug	Probably compatible
Ciprofloxacin	C	Avoid: potential toxicity to cartilage	Limited human data Probably compatible
Corticosteroids	C	Low risk: possible small risk of cleft palate, adrenal insufficiency, premature rupture of membranes	Compatible
Cyclosporine	C	Low risk	Limited human data Potential toxicity
Fish oil supplements	—	Low risk Possibly beneficial	No human data

(continued)

Table 17-1. Medications Used in the Treatment of IBD:
Recommendations for Pregnancy and Breastfeeding (continued)

Drug	Food and Drug Administration Category	Recommendations for Pregnancy	Breastfeeding
Infliximab	B	Limited human data, low risk Crosses placenta and detectable in infant after birth	No evidence of transfer Likely compatible
Mesalamine	B (except Asacol, C)	Low risk. Asacol has Dibutyl Phthalate in coating. Teratogenic in animals at high doses. No evidence of harm in humans.	Limited human data Potential diarrhea
Methotrexate	X	Contraindicated: teratogenic	Contraindicated
Metronidazole	B	Given limited efficacy in IBD, would avoid in first trimester	Limited human data Potential toxicity
Olsalazine	C	Low risk	Limited human data Potential diarrhea

(continued)

Table 17-1. Medications Used in the Treatment of IBD:
Recommendations for Pregnancy and Breastfeeding (continued)

Drug	Food and Drug Administration Category	Recommendations for Pregnancy	Breastfeeding
Risedronate	C	Limited human data, long half-life	Safety unknown
Rifaximin	C	No human data Animal data report some risk	Safety unknown
Sulfasalazine	B	Low risk Give folate 2 mg/day	Limited human data Potential diarrhea
Tacrolimus	C	Low risk	Limited human data Potential toxicity
Thalidomide	X	Contraindicated: teratogenic	No human data Potential toxicity

*Low risk is defined as "the human pregnancy data do not suggest a significant risk of embryo or fetal harm."

- Methotrexate and thalidomide are absolutely contraindicated.
- Metronidazole and ciprofloxacin are relatively contraindicated. Brief courses of metronidazole for 7 to 10 days may be used in the second and third trimesters. For IBD purposes, given their limited efficacy, they are not advised. Breastfeeding is not recommended.
- 5-aminosalicylates are low risk in pregnancy and breastfeeding. If sulfasalazine is used, folic acid 2 mg/day should be given. Sulfasalazine is not known to cause kernicterus in the breastfed infant.
- Prednisone is considered low risk during pregnancy and can be used for disease flares. Its use has been associated with a risk of gestational diabetes and a theoretical risk of adrenal insufficiency in the infant. Use in the first trimester is associated with a small risk of cleft palate. Breastfeeding is allowed.
- Azathioprine (AZA) and 6-mercaptopurine (6-MP) use during pregnancy is controversial. The majority of data in IBD suggest they pose low risk in pregnancy. The risks to the mother of flaring should be balanced against the theoretical risk to the fetus. Breastfeeding can be considered, as levels in breast milk and the newborn are negligible. To minimize exposure, breastfeeding should be avoided for 4 hours after ingestion of 6-MP/AZA, though even during this period, exposure is very low.
- Cyclosporine is likely safer than colectomy in the gravid UC patient with severe, steroid-refractory disease. Fortunately, the need for cyclosporine in this setting is rare.

- The anti-tumor necrosis factor agents—infliximab, adalimumab, and certolizumab—are considered low risk and can be used in pregnancy and breastfeeding.
  - Infliximab and adalimumab are immunoglobulin G subclass 1 antibodies and therefore can cross the placenta highly efficiently in the third trimester and can be detected in the infant for up to 6 months after birth.
  - If the mother is in disease remission, it is recommended that the last medication dose be given at about 30-weeks gestation to minimize exposure to the infant.
  - If the infant has detectable infliximab levels, live virus vaccines (rotavirus) should not be given. As adalimumab levels cannot be checked, live virus vaccines should not be given for the first 6 months to infants whose mothers have received this agent.
  - Certolizumab is a Fab' fragment and has very minimal placental transfer by passive diffusion. It can be continued throughout pregnancy, and vaccination schedules do not need to be altered.

What is the effect of smoking in pregnant women with IBD?

- Smoking has been shown to increase relapse rates and decrease response to medications for Crohn's disease.
- For the health of the fetus (and the mother), the mother should be encouraged to stop smoking.

Do pregnant IBD patients have to have a cesarean section?

- In general, IBD patients can have a normal spontaneous vaginal delivery unless obstetric indications suggest a cesarean section.
- A patient with active perianal disease should have a cesarean section.
- A patient with an ileal pouch–anal anastomosis can deliver vaginally without harming the pouch. However, many surgeons recommend cesarean section, as anal sphincter function is critical in these patients and may be compromised by a vaginal delivery either immediately or in the future.

III. TESTS AND ASSESSMENTS TO ORDER

- Physical examination
  - The patient with an ileostomy may develop obstruction, herniation, or other complications and should be examined regularly for this.
  - Perianal disease should be ruled out prior to delivery.
- Laboratory studies
  - Anemia should be monitored.
  - Given a woman's changing metabolism during pregnancy, patients on 6-MP/AZA or biologics during pregnancy should have a complete blood cell count and liver function tests at least every 2 months.
  - If the mother received infliximab, the infant's infliximab levels should be documented to be undetectable prior to any live virus administration during the first 6 months of life.

- Endoscopy and radiology
  - Endoscopy for IBD is not usually needed during pregnancy. If the patient has severe symptoms and the role of IBD is unclear, an unsedated flexible sigmoidoscopy can be performed safely.
  - Computed tomography scans should be avoided during pregnancy unless absolutely necessary.
  - Magnetic resonance imaging (without gadolinium, a teratogen, in the first trimester) can be performed if needed to assess bowel disease activity.
  - Ultrasound should be performed frequently to monitor for evidence of intrauterine growth retardation.

Suggested Readings

Carter JD, Ladhani A, Ricca LR, Valeriano J, Vasey FB. A safety assessment of tumor necrosis factor antagonists during pregnancy: a review of the Food and Drug Administration database. *J Rheumatol.* 2009;36(3):635-641.

Cleary BJ, Kallén B. Early pregnancy azathioprine use and pregnancy outcomes. *Birth Defects Res A Clin Mol Teratol.* 2009;85(7):647-654.

Kwan LY, Mahadevan U. Inflammatory bowel disease and pregnancy: an update. *Expert Rev Clin Immunol.* 2010;6(4): 643-657.

Nørgård B, Hundborg HH, Jacobsen BA, Nielsen GL, Fonager K. Disease activity in pregnant women with Crohn's disease and birth outcomes: a regional Danish cohort study. *Am J Gastroenterol.* 2007;102(9):1947-1954.

18

The Elderly Patient

Matthew J. Hamilton, MD

The number of patients older than the age of 60 with IBD is increasing as our population becomes older. With regard to disease onset, recent epidemiologic studies have shown that after the initial peak in the second and third decades, the incidence of IBD into the seventh decade remains fairly constant. Establishing the diagnosis of IBD in the elderly patient is a greater challenge than in younger patients because of the longer differential diagnosis, the misconception about the disease prevalence in this population, and the likelihood of an atypical presentation. Careful history taking, examination, and diagnostic studies will help differentiate IBD from other entities that can mimic its various manifestations. Elderly patients who have a diagnosis of IBD are managed in a similar manner to their younger counterparts with regard to induction and maintenance of remission.

Dubinsky M, Friedman S.
Pocket Guide to IBD, Second Edition (pp 125-132).
© 2011 SLACK Incorporated

I. CONDITIONS TO CONSIDER

- Ischemic colitis
- Infectious colitis (*Salmonella, Shigella, Campylobacter, Yersinia, Escherichia coli O157:H7,* cytomegalovirus)
- *Clostridium difficile*–associated colitis
- Diverticular-associated colitis
- Microscopic colitis
- Radiation-induced colitis
- Malignancy and gastrointestinal side effects of chemotherapy
- Medications, particularly nonsteroidal anti-inflammatory drugs (NSAIDs)

II. QUESTIONS TO ASK

Does the patient have an established diagnosis of IBD, or is this a new diagnosis?

- If this is a new diagnosis, other conditions (see "Conditions to Consider") need to be considered and appropriately evaluated.
- In the patient with established IBD and flare of symptoms, a detailed history is necessary to identify potential precipitants (eg, stopping or decreasing IBD medications, antibiotic usage, co-existing gastrointestinal infection).

How severe are the symptoms?

- Have a low threshold to hospitalize the elderly patient. Although response to IBD therapy is similar to that in the younger population, comorbid conditions such as coronary artery disease, hypertension, peripheral vascular disease, and diabetes result in higher morbidity and mortality. Elderly patients at home may find it difficult to take medicines and maintain nutrition and hydration. Reduced mobility may lead to incontinence and falls.

- As with any other condition in elderly patients, be aware of atypical symptoms and signs in IBD. For instance, dehydration, fever, ileus, or pain may manifest as a change in mental status. Coexistent *C difficile* may present solely as leukocytosis.

Is the patient taking NSAIDs or other medications?

- Elderly patients, for a variety of reasons, take NSAIDs at a higher rate than the younger population. It is important to elicit the use of this potential colitis precipitant in every elderly patient with IBD.
- Current or recent use of antibiotics is also common in the elderly patient and may explain an increase in diarrhea by direct (eg, alteration of bowel microflora, carbohydrate maldigestion) or indirect (eg, *C difficile*) mechanisms.

III. IBD MEDICATIONS APPROPRIATE FOR THE ELDERLY PATIENT

- Oral aminosalicylates are well tolerated in patients with ulcerative colitis (UC) and in patients with Crohn's colitis.

- Antibiotics, particularly metronidazole, may be useful in the treatment of Crohn's disease, but patients should be monitored for side effects such as peripheral neuropathy.
- Elderly patients may have difficulty with suppositories or enemas because of decreased sphincter tone and/or rectal compliance. Rectal foam preparations may be more suitable.
- The side effect profiles and efficacy of azathioprine and 6-mercaptopurine for disease maintenance likely are similar in elderly and younger patients.
- Recent evidence suggests that there is probably no difference in the safety or efficacy of anti-tumor necrosis factor biologic medications when used in elderly patients compared to younger patients.
- Corticosteroids are equally effective at inducing remission in the elderly and the younger patient with IBD. However, many of the known side effects are more problematic in the elderly population, and therefore steroid use must be with caution. Patients should be monitored for diabetes and hyperglycemia, congestive heart failure, hypertension, osteoporosis, cataracts, glaucoma, psychosis, and various infections.
- Always be aware of drug interactions in the elderly patient.

IV. Surgical Considerations

- The decision to operate on the elderly patient with IBD should not be delayed.
- Predictors of adverse postoperative outcome include pre-existing health status, presence of comorbidities, severity of the acute attack, and the need for emergent surgery.

- Elderly patients suffer more postoperative cardiac and respiratory complications and have longer mean postoperative hospital stays.
- Ileal pouch–anal anastomosis may result in more erectile dysfunction, fecal incontinence, and diarrhea in the elderly patient.
- There is no significant difference in the frequency of anastomotic leaks, incidence of pouchitis, or pouch failure in elderly patients compared to younger patients.

V. TESTS AND ASSESSMENTS TO ORDER

- Physical examination
  - Pay particular attention to vital signs in the elderly patient, including blood pressure to detect the presence of orthostatic hypotension. In addition, the patient's weight should be charted.
  - Note the patient's general appearance, skin turgor, presence of temporal wasting, and mental status. Perform a careful abdominal examination.
- Laboratory studies
  - Complete blood cell count
  - Anemia-related studies such as an iron panel
  - Inflammatory markers
  - Serum creatinine when certain medications or radiologic studies are being considered
  - Electrolytes when there is a history of diarrhea and/or vomiting
  - Liver function tests
  - Stool cultures and stool tests for *C difficile* in patients with new or worsened diarrhea with or without rectal bleeding and abdominal pain

- An abdominal computed tomography scan is helpful in assessing the severity and extent of colitis in patients with IBD and can also detect other acute-onset forms of colitis such as ischemia, diverticulitis, and infection.
- Colonoscopy will often help to distinguish IBD from other conditions based on the location and appearance of the disease (eg, a new area of edematous mucosa and friability at the splenic flexure may suggest ischemia). Colonoscopy is necessary to rule out colonic malignancy in the elderly patient.
- Directed biopsies during colonoscopy in normal and abnormal areas, in addition to providing key clinical information, will often allow the pathologist to make the diagnosis. For example, a patient with suspected diverticular-associated colitis should have biopsies in the inflamed segment of colon as well as the normal-appearing rectum. The pathologist should be alerted to the fact that the endoscopic inflammation exists only in the area of diverticulosis.

VI. COLON CANCER AND IBD IN THE ELDERLY PATIENT

- The most important risk factors for UC- and Crohn's colitis–associated dysplasia and cancer are disease extent, duration, and severity. The appropriate guidelines for screening patients with IBD for colon cancer pertain also to the elderly patient and should be followed.
- The incidence of sporadic colon polyps and colorectal cancer increases with age.
- With advances in IBD therapy, patients are keeping their colons longer and therefore are

at increased risk of dysplasia-associated cancer and sporadic malignant disease.

SUGGESTED READINGS

Ananthakrishnan AN, McGinley EL, Binion DG. Inflammatory bowel disease in the elderly is associated with worse outcomes: a national study of hospitalizations. *Inflamm Bowel Dis*. 2009;15(2):182-189.

Chevillotte-Maillard H, Ornetti P, Mistrih R, et al. Survival and safety of treatment with infliximab in the elderly population. *Rheumatology*. 2005;44(5):695-696.

Loftus CG, Loftus EV Jr, Harmsen WS, et al. Update on the incidence and prevalence of Crohn's disease and ulcerative colitis in Olmsted County, Minnesota,1940-2000. *Inflamm Bowel Dis*. 2007;13(3):254-261.

Shivananda S, Lennard-Jones J, Logan R, et al. Incidence of inflammatory bowel disease across Europe: is there a difference between north and south? Results of the European Collaborative Study on Inflammatory Bowel Disease (EC-IBD). *Gut*. 1996;39(5):690-697.

Travis S. Is IBD different in the elderly? *Inflamm Bowel Dis*. 2008;14 Suppl 2:S12-S13.

SECTION V

SPECIAL
CONSIDERATIONS

9

Colorectal Cancer

David T. Rubin, MD, FACG, AGAF

Patients with chronic IBD of the colon or rectum have an increased risk for colorectal cancer (CRC). Although this is a rare complication of IBD, the morbidity and mortality associated with this complication have been well described, and prevention strategies have been developed. The patient newly diagnosed with IBD is faced with a bewildering array of emotional and physical problems; learning that this disease may also cause bowel cancer invariably causes anxiety and fear. These feelings should be addressed by the health care provider and may be ameliorated by helping the patient understand his or her individual risks, describing the relative rarity of this complication, and engaging the patient in effective prevention strategies.

I. CONDITIONS TO CONSIDER

- Chronic ulcerative colitis (UC)
- Chronic Crohn's colitis

Dubinsky M, Friedman S.
Pocket Guide to IBD, Second Edition (pp 135-148).
© 2011 SLACK Incorporated

II. Questions to Ask

What is the risk of colon cancer in patients with IBD?

- The majority of studies and published evidence regarding colorectal cancer in IBD have involved patients with UC, although the association in patients with Crohn's disease of the colon has been increasingly reported and is now accepted as well.

- A 2001 meta-analysis of previous studies demonstrated that the overall prevalence of CRC in patients with UC is approximately 3.6% and that the cumulative incidence increases related to increasing duration of disease from approximately 2% after 10 years of disease to approximately 20% by 30 years of disease. Most experienced clinicians, however, believe that these calculations are higher than the actual rates and may reflect publication and referral biases. In fact, more recent evidence suggests that the cumulative incidence of CRC in UC may be less than half of these older values.

How does colon cancer develop in patients with IBD?

- Colorectal cancer in patients with IBD is believed to arise from precancerous dysplasia, therefore, similar to the practice of identifying precancerous polyps in the approach to cancer prevention in the non-IBD population, dysplasia is used as a marker of risk and a target for identification in IBD.
  - Dysplasia in IBD is characterized as indefinite, low-grade dysplasia (LGD) or high-grade dysplasia (HGD).

- The different grades of dysplasia are associated with different risks of *concurrent* adenocarcinoma found at colectomy and with different risks of *progression* to higher-grade neoplasia (including adenocarcinoma) if the patient keeps his or her colon and is followed over time.
- This predictive information has lead to an approach of prevention focused on the identification of dysplasia and the use of proctocolectomy as a secondary prevention strategy.

What are the individual risks for colon cancer in patients with IBD?

- Knowing the patient's individual risks for CRC can aid in cancer prevention in patients with IBD.
- Known risk factors for dysplasia and CRC in patients with chronic UC (and probably Crohn's colitis) include those that are immutable:
  - Longer duration of disease
  - Greater extent of colonic involvement
  - Family history of CRC (independent of a family history of IBD)
  - Co-existing primary sclerosing cholangitis (PSC)
  - Younger age at diagnosis
- Risk factors that are potentially modifiable, and in theory may therefore be controlled to lower risk, include the following:
  - A greater degree of histologic inflammation of the bowel
  - The development of pseudopolyps
  - "Backwash ileitis," in which the small intestine adjacent to the ileocecal valve is exposed to inflammatory "backwash" through the ileocecal valve

- Both pseudopolyps and backwash ileitis may in fact be simply surrogate markers of more extensive colitis.

How can the development of colon cancer be prevented in IBD patients?

- It is believed that most CRC in patients with IBD can be prevented if both the patient and the caregiver are educated about risks and adhere to published guidelines.
- Prevention of CRC in patients with IBD requires risk stratification of the patient based on the compounded risk factors as well as a combination of surveillance colonoscopy and appropriately timed proctocolectomy.
- There may be benefits from chemoprevention with some therapeutic agents (described later in this chapter).

Why do we need surveillance guidelines?

- The appearance of polyps in the non-IBD patient, which are typically sporadic, is different than in the patient with chronic colitis. In patients with chronic colitis, there is believed to be a "field effect" in which the entire involved colon is at risk and therefore may develop multifocal neoplastic changes.
- Dysplasia in patients with IBD may occur in the flat mucosa and not be readily visible to the endoscopist.
- Guidelines were developed to account for these challenges and include systematic sampling of the at-risk mucosa by random and targeted biopsies.

What are the IBD colon cancer surveillance guidelines?

- The guidelines recommend colonoscopy after approximately 8 years of disease and repeated colonoscopy every 1 to 3 years thereafter (interval is determined based on compounded risk factors as well as findings of the last examination), with random biopsies looking for dysplasia and additional biopsies of any polypoid structures, strictures, or masses.
- The exception is the patient with PSC, in whom surveillance colonoscopy should begin at the time of diagnosis and be repeated annually (Table 19-1).

Why should we educate patients about surveillance colonoscopy?

- Although patients may resist the idea of regularly scheduled colonoscopies, it is important to educate them that surveillance colonoscopy is believed to be an effective prevention strategy.
- The goal is to identify precancerous dysplasia and, when CRC has already developed, to find it at an earlier stage.
- Patients undergoing surveillance colonoscopy who develop CRC are more likely to have CRC at a lower stage and have an associated improved survival than those who do not undergo surveillance.

Table 19-1. Guidelines for
Cancer Prevention in IBD

1. UC or Crohn's colitis (without primary sclerosing cholangitis, PSC) for >8 years: surveillance colonoscopy with 3 or 4 biopsies every 10 cm, for a total of approximately 33 biopsies. Target raised lesions, mucosal irregularity that is distinct from surrounding mucosa, strictures, and masses. Polypectomy when endoscopically distinct raised lesions are identified. Separate biopsies around the lesion to look for a localized field effect. Repeat every 1 to 3 years depending on compounded risks. If the patient has PSC, see #4. Chromoendoscopy with dye spraying consistently demonstrated greater sensitivity to detect dysplasia than white light examinations. However, its routine use in surveillance colonoscopy has not been defined and cannot yet be broadly endorsed.

2. If high-grade dysplasia is identified, confirm by review of a second pathologist. If confirmed, recommend proctocolectomy. If low-grade dysplasia is identified, discuss proctocolectomy and refer for surgical consultation.

3. Some patients with focal and visible low-grade dysplasia may be followed with a more intensive surveillance approach, but this will require both physician and provider active participation. Consider referral to specialty centers for assistance.

4. Encourage adherence to 5-aminosalicylate therapy (≥ 1.2 g/day) for maintenance as well as for proposed chemopreventive properties. If the patient has PSC, start surveillance at the time of diagnosis and continue yearly. In addition, patients with PSC and UC should be on ursodeoxycholic acid 300 mg twice daily.

If LGD is found, what is the risk of concurrent HGD and carcinoma?

- Because random biopsies are used to screen for dysplasia in the flat lining of the colon, additional higher-grade lesions may be identified at the time of colectomy.
- In fact, concurrent adenocarcinoma is found in the colons of 19% of patients who undergo colectomy for a finding of LGD and 67% of patients who undergo colectomy for a finding of HGD.
- Therefore, the diagnosis of HGD confirmed by more than one pathologist should always be treated by proctocolectomy, and the diagnosis of LGD should prompt a surgical consultation and careful discussion of risks and benefits of proctocolectomy versus increased surveillance.

Does LGD progress to a more sinister lesion, and should the colon be removed prior to progression?

- Recent work has shown LGD that is not removed may progress to a higher grade or to cancer in 20% to 50% of cases during the subsequent 5 years.
- However, an evolving understanding about the identification of dysplasia and the removal of polypoid lesions suggests that a carefully selected subset of patients may be followed with more intensive surveillance examinations.

What is the evolving role for chromoendoscopy in IBD cancer prevention?

- Existing high-definition white-light colonoscopes are able to visualize dysplastic lesions in most patients, and the effectiveness in the identification of dysplasia has been increased with the addition of chromoendoscopic techniques with dye spraying of methylene blue.
- Currently, chromoendoscopy is recommended to aid in the identification of borders of lesions and for enhancement of segments of colon in which dysplasia has been identified or is suspected. A more detailed rationale and approach is evolving (Table 19-2).

What is the role of chemoprevention—using medications in patients with IBD?

- A number of agents have been proposed to prevent the development of dysplasia and CRC in patients with long-standing colitis.
  - The gallstone-dissolution agent ursodeoxycholic acid (URSO) is used to treat other biliary diseases but also has been shown to prevent dysplasia and cancer in patients with IBD and PSC at doses of 300 mg twice daily, so this agent is now recommended independent of its therapeutic benefits for PSC alone. It remains unknown whether URSO will be helpful in IBD patients who do not have PSC.
  - 5-aminosalicylic acid (5-ASA), a mainstay of therapy for patients with UC, has been shown

Table 19-2. Suggested Rationale and Approach to Chromoendoscopy for the Detection of Dysplasia in IBD

1. This technique is not yet standardized and is not yet in society guidelines.

2. However, it is acknowledged that chromoendoscopy increases the detection of dysplasia in IBD patients.

3. Methylene blue or indigo carmine dye spraying should be used; narrow-band imaging has not been demonstrated to have specific benefit in this situation.

4. It is essential that the patient has had a pristine colonic preparation and has adequate colonic stasis during a quality chromoendoscopy examination. Some investigators have described using glucagon or other bowel relaxants to assist in visualization.

5. Dye is administered in a segmental fashion after reaching the colon and completing inspection of the ileum (when appropriate). A dye-spraying catheter or 60-cc syringe with diluted dye (1:10 cc methylene blue) can be used. *Note:* Methylene blue is absorbed into the cytoplasm of cells and therefore adheres more easily to specific nongravity-dependent portions of the colon. Indigo carmine does not have this property, so repositioning the patient to allow for shifting of fluid may be necessary.

6. Adequate power washing and spraying are used as an adjunct to remove debris and enhance visualization.

7. Tattooing of suspicious areas should be performed, especially if there is a possibility of subsequent examinations.

8. Clear labeling of all specimen jars and separation of concerning findings from surrounding mucosal biopsies will assist the pathologist in diagnosing any findings.

to have unique chemopreventive properties for both dysplasia and CRC in chronic UC. In a meta-analysis of cohort and case-control studies, use of 5-ASA at doses of 1.2 g/day or greater reduced the risk of dysplasia and cancer by approximately 50%.

○ More recent studies that actually adjust for the degree of bowel inflammation suggest that this benefit may be due in part to lower degrees of inflammation. Nonetheless, the efficacy and safety of 5-ASA for treatment of UC and maintenance of remission support a discussion of this potential benefit with patients, both to encourage adherence to maintenance therapy and to stress the importance of enrolling in a cancer prevention program.

○ In patients with multiple risks of neoplasia but whose medical therapy has been escalated beyond 5-ASA, one may consider continuing some dose of 5-ASA for its possible preventive properties.

CONCLUSION

CRC is a recognized but rare complication of IBD. The approach to the patient with UC or Crohn's colitis should include education about risk factors and effective prevention strategies. Enrolling the patient in a proactive prevention program involving education, risk factor identification, colonoscopies and biopsies, and frank discussions and recommendations regarding colectomy is essential to the comprehensive care of these chronic conditions. Advancing technologies have provided some new insights into the possibilities of continuing to follow patients with confirmed dysplasia, but a unified approach to this process is not yet defined.

Suggested Readings

Canavan C, Abrams KR, Mayberry J. Meta-analysis: colorectal and small bowel cancer risk in patients with Crohn's disease. *Aliment Pharmacol Ther*. 2006;23(8):1097-1104.

Choi PM, Nugent FW, Schoetz DJ Jr, et al. Colonoscopic surveillance reduces mortality from colorectal cancer in ulcerative colitis. *Gastroenterology*. 1993;105(2):418-424.

Eaden JA, Abrams KR, Mayberry JF. The risk of colorectal cancer in ulcerative colitis: a meta-analysis. *Gut*. 2001;48(4):526-535.

Gupta RB, Harpaz N, Itzkowitz S, et al. Histologic inflammation is a risk factor for progression to colorectal neoplasia in ulcerative colitis: a cohort study. *Gastroenterology*. 2007;133(4):1099-1105.

Itzkowitz SH, Harpaz N. Diagnosis and management of dysplasia in patients with inflammatory bowel diseases. *Gastroenterology*. 2004;126(6):1634-1648.

Itzkowitz SH, Present DH. Consensus conference: colorectal cancer screening and surveillance in inflammatory bowel disease. *Inflamm Bowel Dis*. 2005;11(3):314-321.

Jess T, Loftus EV Jr, Velayos FS, et al. Risk of intestinal cancer in inflammatory bowel disease: a population-based study from Olmsted County, Minnesota. *Gastroenterology*. 2006;130(4):1039-1046.

Karlén P, Kornfeld D, Broström O, et al. Is colonoscopic surveillance reducing colorectal cancer mortality in ulcerative colitis? A population based case control study [see comments]. *Gut*. 1998;42(5):711-714.

Kiesslich R, Neurath MF. Chromoendoscopy: an evolving standard in surveillance for ulcerative colitis. *Inflamm Bowel Dis*. 2004;10(5):695-696.

Kornbluth A, Sachar DB. Ulcerative colitis practice guidelines in adults (update): American College of Gastroenterology, Practice Parameters Committee. *Am J Gastroenterol*. 2004;99(7):1371-1385.

Marion JF, Waye JD, Present DH, et al. Chromoendoscopy-targeted biopsies are superior to standard colonoscopic surveillance for detecting dysplasia in inflammatory bowel disease patients: a prospective endoscopic trial. *Am J Gastroenterol*. 2008;103(9):2342-2349.

Pardi DS, Loftus EV Jr, Kremers WK, et al. Ursodeoxycholic acid as a chemopreventive agent in patients with ulcerative colitis and primary sclerosing cholangitis. *Gastroenterology.* 2003;124(4):889-893.

Pekow JR, Hetzel JT, Rothe JA, et al. Outcome after surveillance of low-grade and indefinite dysplasia in patients with ulcerative colitis. *Inflamm Bowel Dis.* 2010;16(8):1352-1356.

Riddell R, Goldman H, Ransohoff DF, et al. Dysplasia in inflammatory bowel disease: standardized classification with provisional clinical applications. *Hum Pathol.* 1983;14(11):931-968.

Rubin DT. An updated approach to dysplasia in IBD. *J Gastrointest Surg.* 2008;12(12):2153-2156.

Rubin DT, Kavitt RT. Surveillance for cancer and dysplasia in inflammatory bowel disease. *Gastroenterol Clin North Am.* 2006;35(3):581-604.

Rubin DT, Rothe JA, Hetzel JT, et al. Are dysplasia and colorectal cancer endoscopically visible in patients with ulcerative colitis? *Gastrointest Endosc.* 2007;65(7):998-1004.

Rutter MD, Saunders BP, Schofield G, et al. Pancolonic indigo carmine dye spraying for the detection of dysplasia in ulcerative colitis. *Gut.* 2004;53(2):256-260.

Rutter MD, Saunders BP, Wilkinson KH, et al. Most dysplasia in ulcerative colitis is visible at colonoscopy. *Gastrointest Endosc.* 2004;60(3):334-339.

Rutter MD, Saunders BP, Wilkinson KH, et al. Severity of inflammation is a risk factor for colorectal neoplasia in ulcerative colitis. *Gastroenterology.* 2004;126(2):451-459.

Rutter MD, Saunders BP, Wilkinson KH, et al. Thirty-year analysis of a colonoscopic surveillance program for neoplasia in ulcerative colitis. *Gastroenterology.* 2006;130(4):1030-1038.

Siegel CA, Schwartz LM, Woloshin S, et al. When should ulcerative colitis patients undergo colectomy for dysplasia? Mismatch between patient preferences and physician recommendations. *Inflamm Bowel Dis.* 2010;16(10):1658-1662.

Ullman T, Croog V, Harpaz N, et al. Progression of flat low-grade dysplasia to advanced neoplasia in patients with ulcerative colitis. *Gastroenterology.* 2003;125(5):1311-1319.

Velayos FS, Loftus EV Jr, Jess T, et al. Predictive and protective factors associated with colorectal cancer in ulcerative colitis: a case-control study. *Gastroenterology.* 2006;130(7):1941-1949.

Velayos FS, Terdiman JP, Walsh JM. Effect of 5-aminosalicylate use on colorectal cancer and dysplasia risk: a systematic review and metaanalysis of observational studies. *Am J Gastroenterol.* 2005;100(6):1345-1353.

Zisman TL, Rubin DT. Colorectal cancer and dysplasia in inflammatory bowel disease. *World J Gastroenterol.* 2008;14(17):2662-2669.

20

Nutritional Issues

Erin Feldman, RD, CSP

There are many theories about food and its relationship to IBD; however, few standards of care exist for the use of nutritional therapies in IBD. We do know that excellent nutrition is essential to improve overall health in patients with Crohn's disease (CD) and ulcerative colitis (UC).

I. CONDITIONS TO CONSIDER

- Weight loss
- Malnutrition
- Malabsorption of nutrients
- Lactose intolerance

Dubinsky M, Friedman S.
Pocket Guide to IBD, Second Edition (pp 149-156).
© 2011 SLACK Incorporated

II. QUESTIONS TO ASK

What factors contribute to malnutrition in patients with IBD?

- Decreased nutrient intake secondary to loss of appetite and abdominal pain
- Malabsorption/gastrointestinal losses with associated vitamin and mineral deficiencies
- An overly restricted diet

How can the malnutrition be reversed?

- *Consumption of adequate calories.* Most adult patients with IBD require 25 to 35 calories/kg of ideal body weight (IBW) and 1 to 1.5 g/kg of IBW of protein per day.
- *Frequent meals throughout the day.* Eating frequent meals throughout the day can help the patient meet his or her nutritional requirements of calories, protein, vitamins, and minerals.
- *Supplementation with oral nutritional products.* If it is impossible for the patient to consume adequate nutrition with food alone, supplementation is necessary. A concentrated formula may be indicated if a patient requires a large amount of supplemental calories (1.5 calories/cc).
- *Vitamin/mineral supplementation.* Patients with IBD are at risk for developing multiple vitamin and mineral deficiencies, most often secondary to inadequate intake of nutrients (Table 20-1).

Table 20-1. Vitamin and Mineral Supplementation in Patients With IBD

Vitamin/Mineral	Possible Cause of Deficiency	Supplemental Dose	Food Sources	Comments
Folic acid	Sulfasalazine and methotrexate may alter absorption and metabolism	1 mg/day	Leafy green vegetables, citrus fruits and juices, dried beans and peas, and enriched grain products	Folic acid may also play a role in colon cancer protection
Vitamin D	Increased disease activity	800 IU/day for active disease and during corticosteroid treatment	Fish (tuna, salmon, mackerel), fish liver oils, and fortified dairy products	Vitamin D deficiency contributes to low bone mineral density and osteoporosis; most common deficiency in Crohn's disease.
Vitamin B$_{12}$	Ileal disease, resection of the ileum, or bacterial overgrowth	RDA: 2.4 µg/day Supplemental doses vary based on route of administration	Animal products such as fish, meat, poultry, eggs, milk and milk products, and fortified breakfast cereals	

(continued)

Table 20-1. Vitamin and Mineral Supplementation in Patients With IBD (continued)

Vitamin/Mineral	Possible Cause of Deficiency	Supplemental Dose	Food Sources	Comments
Calcium	Corticosteroids can decrease the absorption of calcium	1200 to 1500 mg/day	Milk, yogurt, cheese, Chinese cabbage, kale, and broccoli	Calcium is important for maintaining strong bones
Zinc	Severe diarrhea, enteric fistulas, and moderate disease activity	25 to 50 mg/day	Oysters, red meat, poultry, beans, nuts, crab, lobster, whole grains, fortified breakfast cereals, and dairy products	The body has no specialized zinc storage system
Iron	Decreased intake, increased losses, and/or decreased absorption	2 to 3 mg/kg/day	Red meats, fish, poultry, lentils, beans, and iron-fortified foods	Vitamin C helps to increase absorption of iron

RDA indicates recommended daily allowance; IU, international units.

Does the patient require an alternative form of nutritional support?

- An alternative form of nutritional support is required if the patient is unable to consume adequate nutrition orally and experiences weight loss or failure to gain weight.
- Enteral nutrition (by mouth/nasogastric/by gastrostomy) can be used as supplemental nutrition to the patient's oral diet or as the sole source of nutrition therapy when oral intake is very poor or disease activity is severe. Studies have shown that nutritional therapy using enteral products may result in disease remission rates similar to when corticosteroids are used. Compliance can become an issue when enteral nutrition is used as the sole source of nutrition.
- Total parenteral nutrition (TPN) is used when the enteral route cannot be used or when bowel rest is necessary. Few studies have explored the therapeutic effect of TPN on IBD, although based on the studies that have been completed, TPN appears to have more of a benefit for patients with CD than those with UC (Table 20-2).

Table 20-2. Nutritional Therapy Recommendations

• Consumption of adequate calories to maintain a healthy weight or promote weight gain if indicated
• Use of supplemental calories, orally or enterally, based on the patient's needs
• Use of total parental nutrition if the gastrointestinal tract cannot be used for feeding
• Daily multivitamin, along with additional supplemental vitamins and minerals, as needed (based on chemistry levels, drug therapy, and clinical findings)
• Avoidance of unnecessary restrictions in the diet to ensure optimal nutritional intake

Should patients with IBD avoid dairy products?

- Lactose intolerance has not been proven to affect patients with IBD more than the US population in general.
- The prevalence of lactose intolerance is greater in patients with CD affecting the small bowel than in patients with Crohn's colitis or UC.
- Symptoms of lactose intolerance include diarrhea, nausea, vomiting, abdominal cramps, bloating, and early satiety, which are all symptoms that may be present with IBD. If there is question about whether a patient is lactose intolerant, it is recommended to remove dairy products from the diet and monitor for improvement in symptoms. If no change is seen, dairy is slowly added back into the diet. Hydrogen breath testing is another way to test for lactose intolerance.

Is a low-residue diet recommended?

- A low-residue diet may be recommended for certain IBD patients on a temporary basis. The diet is usually followed until the inflammation responds to medical treatment.
- Patients with strictures or areas of narrowing may benefit from following a low-residue diet long term to minimize abdominal pain, decrease other symptoms, and prevent obstructions from occurring.
- Patients following a low-residue diet should avoid foods high in fiber, especially raw fruits and vegetables, seeds, nuts, and popcorn.

Is there a role for omega-3 and omega-6 fatty acids?

- The omega-3 fatty acids eicosapentaenoic acid and docosahexaenoic acid, both found in fish oil, have been shown to have anti-inflammatory properties and may decrease disease activity and the rate of relapse in patients with CD who are in remission.
- Omega-6 fatty acids (found in safflower oil, corn oil, walnuts, and oils found in most snack foods) may have proinflammatory properties when consumed in large amounts.
- It is hypothesized that following a Mediterranean-style diet including fish and olive oil is beneficial for patients with IBD. Additional studies are needed to clarify dosage and duration of treatment.

Do probiotics help patients with IBD?

- The gut flora plays an important role in maintaining normal intestinal function. In IBD, a disturbance of the flora is seen. Probiotics may improve the microbial balance in the intestine. Further studies are needed to answer questions related to the benefit of probiotics and the dosage, duration, and frequency of treatment with probiotics.

III. Tests and Assessments to Order

- Laboratory studies
  - Complete blood cell count
  - Serum albumin
  - Serum electrolytes
  - Folic acid and vitamin B_{12}
  - Serum iron, total iron-binding capacity, and ferritin
  - Serum calcium, magnesium, phosphorus
  - Alkaline phosphatase (surrogate marker for zinc deficiency)
  - Vitamin D
- Additional tests if growth failure or significant malnutrition is present
  - Vitamin A, vitamin E, prothrombin time, and zinc
  - Bone age (if growth is impaired)

Suggested Readings

Akobeng AK, Thomas AG. Enteral nutrition for maintenance of remission in Crohn's disease. *Cochrane Database Syst Rev.* 2007;18(3):CD005984.

Mijac DD, Jankovic GL, Jorga J, et al. Nutritional status in patients with active inflammatory bowel disease: prevalence of malnutrition and methods for routine nutritional assessment. *Eur J Intern Med.* 2010;21(4):315-319.

Yamamoto T, Nakahigashi M, Saniabadi AR. Review article: diet and inflammatory bowel disease—epidemiology and treatment. *Aliment Pharmacol Ther.* 2009;30(2):99-112.

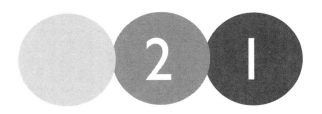

Osteoporosis

Edward V. Loftus Jr, MD

Osteoporosis, or "thinning of the bones," is a concern among many women, especially those who are experiencing or have experienced menopause. Osteoporosis increases one's susceptibility to developing fractures of the bones in the wrist, ribs, vertebral spine, and hips, often with minimal trauma. Osteoporosis accounts for 1.5 million fractures and results in more than $13 billion in medical costs in the United States annually. It is estimated that more than 5 million US citizens have osteoporosis, and more than 21 million have a precursor condition called osteopenia. Although postmenopausal white women are at highest risk for osteoporosis and osteopenia, these conditions are occurring with increasing frequency in men and non-white women.

RISK FACTORS

Numerous studies show that patients with IBD, especially Crohn's disease (CD), are at increased risk for osteoporosis and osteopenia. Some population-based estimates

Dubinsky M, Friedman S.
Pocket Guide to IBD, Second Edition (pp 157-164).
© 2011 SLACK Incorporated

suggest that osteoporosis may occur in as many as 1 in 7 patients with CD, while osteopenia may occur in as many as 45%. No single reason explains why IBD is a risk factor for osteoporosis.

Possible explanations for osteoporosis in patients with IBD include the following:

- Corticosteroids such as prednisone have been known for years to have powerful effects on bone metabolism. Studies show that decreased bone density and increased fracture risk may occur within a few months of starting steroids. Even low-dose prednisone (5 mg daily) usage has been associated with increased fracture risk.
- Other drugs such as cyclosporine and methotrexate may reduce bone density slightly.
- IBD itself, especially CD, may be a risk factor. Low bone densities have been noted in newly diagnosed patients, even before they have received corticosteroids. It is thought that perhaps elevated levels of circulating inflammatory cytokines have negative effects on bone formation and resorption.
- Patients with CD with small bowel involvement, or with a history of small bowel resections, may not properly absorb calcium and/or vitamin D.
- Many patients with IBD have a low body mass index, which is an independent risk factor for osteoporosis.
- Cigarette smoking is a risk factor for osteoporosis, and many patients with CD have a history of former or current smoking.
- It is important to note that the most important risk factors for osteoporosis in the general population—older age, female gender, and low body mass index—are also the most important predictors of osteoporosis in the IBD population.

Low bone mineral density does not necessarily corre-
late exactly with fracture risk, so it is important to determine whether patients with IBD have an increased risk of
fracture. Most studies of fracture risk in IBD suggest that
patients with IBD are anywhere from 15% to 45% more
likely than the general population to develop an osteoporotic fracture (hip, spine, wrist, or ribs). In most, but not
all, studies, the fracture risk seems slightly higher in CD.
It is interesting to note that the smaller studies (ie, a few
hundred patients) have not demonstrated an increased
fracture risk, while the larger studies (ie, a few thousand
patients) have. In other words, we can reassure our patients that although their fracture risk is increased, it may
not be as high as previously thought.

WHO TO SCREEN

If the risk of fracture is elevated (but not "sky-high") in
IBD, how do we decide which patients should be tested
for osteoporosis? Blanket screening of all patients with
IBD would probably result in unnecessary testing. The
IBD patients most at risk for fracture are postmenopausal
women, patients with low body mass index, and those
receiving steroids. Guidelines from several gastroen-
terologic societies recommend that dual-energy x-ray
absorptiometry (DEXA) scanning be performed in IBD
patients with one or more of the following risk factors:
age >60 years, low body mass index, heavy smoking
history, postmenopausal, steroid treatment for at least
3 months, recurrent courses of steroids, and a history of
prior fractures.

FRACTURE RISK ASSESSMENT

The results of a DEXA scan are usually given as a
T-score. The T-score indicates the standard deviation from
the mean peak bone mass in the general population. In

other words, a score of −3 indicates that the patient's bone density is 3 standard deviations below the mean, while a score of 0 indicates a bone density exactly at the mean. A patient is considered to have osteoporosis if the T-score in the lumbar spine, hip, or wrist is below −2.5, while osteopenia is defined as a T-score between −1 and −2.5.

TREATMENT OF OSTEOPOROSIS

The following measures can be used to treat IBD-associated osteoporosis (Figure 21-1).

- Lifestyle modifications, such as regular exercise and cessation of cigarette smoking, should be encouraged.
- Elemental calcium intake should be at least 1200 mg/day. For patients who do not ingest this amount of calcium in their diet, a calcium carbonate or calcium citrate supplement should be recommended.
- Vitamin D intake should range from 400 to 800 international units daily. Higher levels may be required in patients with malabsorption or vitamin D deficiency. (Such deficiency should be corrected prior to treatment with a bisphosphonate.)
- Strong consideration should be given to the use of IBD medications that allow steroid-dependent patients to wean successfully off steroids. Examples include azathioprine, 6-mercaptopurine, methotrexate, and anti-tumor necrosis factor inhibitors.
- Estrogen seems to be falling out of favor after one study showed that the risks (increase in cardiovascular events and breast cancers) outweigh the benefits of combined estrogen-progestin therapy. However, selective estrogen-receptor modulators

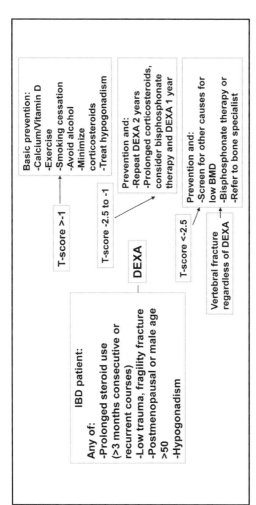

Figure 21-1. Recommendations for managing osteoporosis. BMD indicates bone mineral density; DEXA, dual-energy X-ray absorptiometry. (Adapted from Bernstein CN, Leslie WD, Leboff MS. AGA technical review on osteoporosis in gastrointestinal diseases. *Gastroenterology.* 2003;124(3):795-841.)

such as raloxifene may increase bone density and reduce fracture risk, but not at the cost of an increase in breast cancers.

- Bisphosphonates, which block bone resorption, can be administered. Two oral bisphosphonates, alendronate and risedronate, which can be given on either a daily or a weekly basis, have been shown to increase vertebral and femoral neck bone density and reduce vertebral and hip fractures for both postmenopausal and glucocorticoid-induced osteoporosis. In addition, risedronate prevents bone loss in patients receiving corticosteroids. Ibandronate can be given orally on a daily or monthly basis, or given intravenously (IV) every 3 months, and has also been approved by the Food and Drug Administration (FDA) for the prevention and treatment of postmenopausal osteoporosis. It has been shown to increase bone mineral density and decrease fracture risk with a superiority for the IV formulation. Gastrointestinal side effects, including esophagitis, may occasionally occur with oral administration of any of these medications, necessitating other treatment alternatives.

- Pamidronate, 60 mg IV every 3 to 6 months, has been used by some physicians to deliver bisphosphonates for those who cannot tolerate oral preparations. Zoledronic acid (5 mg IV/year) is FDA-approved for the prevention and treatment of both postmenopausal and glucocorticoid-induced osteoporosis, as well as the treatment of osteoporosis in men.

- Nasal calcitonin-salmon spray has also been shown to be effective for improving bone density and reducing fracture risk in the lumbar spine, primarily in women who are >5 years postmenopausal.

- Recombinant parathyroid hormone, or teriparatide, when administered subcutaneously on a daily basis, can improve bone density and reduce fracture risk significantly. However, because of the observation of osteosarcomas in laboratory rats following the administration of this drug, the FDA has suggested that its use be limited to patients for whom the potential benefits are considered to outweigh the potential risk (ie, those with a previous history of osteoporotic fracture, multiple risk factors, or who have failed or are intolerant to other treatments), and it is contraindicated in children and adolescents.

By following the guidelines presented herein, we can identify patients with IBD at risk for osteoporosis, use a noninvasive screening tool to test them, and then choose an agent to reduce their future risk of fracture. Remember, preventing a complication is always easier than treating one!

Suggested Readings

Bernstein CN. Osteoporosis in patients with inflammatory bowel disease. *Clin Gastroenterol Hepatol.* 2006;4(2):152-166.

Bernstein CN, Leslie WD. Therapy insight: osteoporosis in inflammatory bowel disease—advances and retreats. *Nat Clin Pract Gastroenterol Hepatol.* 2005;2(5):232-239.

Bernstein CN, Leslie WD, Leboff MS. AGA technical review on osteoporosis in gastrointestinal diseases. *Gastroenterology.* 2003;124(3):795-841.

Lichtenstein GR, Sands BE, Pazianas M. Prevention and treatment of osteoporosis in inflammatory bowel disease. *Inflamm Bowel Dis.* 2006;12(8):797-813.

Tilg H, Moschen AR, Kaser A, et al. *Gut, inflammation and osteoporosis: basic and clinical concepts. Gut.* 2008;57(5): 684-694.

22

The Nonadherent Patient

Sunanda V. Kane, MD, MSPH, FACG, FACP, AGAF

Your patient is feeling great and asks you, "Do I really need to take so much medicine? After all, it's been a while (thankfully) since I've had a flare of my disease." What should your response be? It is crucial to emphasize to your patients the importance of continuing their maintenance medications. Here is a partial list why:

- IBD is a chronic, incurable disease, just like diabetes. You would not tell a diabetic to stop taking insulin just because he or she feels well.
- The inflammation in the digestive tract is present even if a patient feels well and will get the better of the patient if he or she lets it. Medications help to slow the inflammatory process and promote healing, which ultimately leads to a decreased risk of potential complications (such as surgery) in the future.

Dubinsky M, Friedman S.
Pocket Guide to IBD, Second Edition (pp 165-168).
© 2011 SLACK Incorporated

- Several studies have shown what even short-term discontinuation of medications can do, especially if the patient has required long courses of steroids in the past.
- Not taking medications can lead to more aggressive flares, which may require steroid therapy, hospitalization, or surgery. The long-term consequences of steroids are well known and include cataract formation, osteoporosis, and poor skin healing.
- A long-term study performed at the University of Chicago showed that patients who were followed for 2 years had a *5-fold* increased risk for a disease flare of ulcerative colitis if they took less than 80% of their prescribed medication over that time period. Those patients who continued on their medications regularly were less likely to have to visit the doctor or to have procedures, and ultimately saved money.
- Two studies have shown that patients taking long-term azathioprine for Crohn's disease are at risk for a flare if they stop taking it, even when they have been well for close to 5 years.
- Another study conducted at the University of Chicago and 5 studies conducted at other institutions have shown that taking certain medicines such as mesalamine may decrease risk for the development of cancer.

Why do patients stop taking their medications? Most physicians do not do a good job explaining to patients the purpose of medications and the importance of their continued use. In addition, patients are sometimes too embarrassed to admit that they do not know what their medications do, that their medications cost too much, or that they are not taking them. Open dialogue between the patient, the physician, and other members of the health care team is the best way to address concerns so that complications can be avoided.

Which patients are more likely to not take their medications? The answer turns out to be those patients who do not have a good support system, including single people and young college students. Males seem to be particularly susceptible to this behavior. How do we as physicians combat this problem? We get others involved, such as our patients' friends and organizations such as the Crohn's and Colitis Foundation of America (CCFA) so that patients do not feel so alone.

Another way to help patients improve their medication-taking behavior is to make things easy for them. Here is a list of ideas.

- When possible, schedule medication doses twice a day or even once a day rather than 3 or 4 times a day.
- Have patients put their pills in several places so that when it is time to take them, they have some available nearby. Taking them "later" often leads to skipped doses.
- Ensure that patients understand what to do if they miss a dose. Do they double up the next dose or just forget about the missed dose? There can be consequences to missing too many doses, and this should be discussed with patients.
- Make sure your patients tell you everything they are taking. You may not agree with some of these preparations, but at least you can then monitor for unwanted or unexpected side effects.
- Encourage your patients to ask questions! If they do not understand what a pill does or what they should expect from it, then they are less likely to take it. If patients are having trouble paying for a medication, discuss generic formulations and patient assistance programs.

Suggested Readings

Higgins PD, Rubin DT, Kaulback K, Schoenfeld PS, Kane SV. Systematic review: impact of non-adherence to 5-ASA products on the frequency and cost of ulcerative colitis flares. *Aliment Pharmacol Ther.* 2009;29(3):247-257.

Kane SV, Aikens J, Huo D, Hanauer SB. Medication adherence is associated with improved outcomes in patients with quiescent ulcerative colitis. *Am J Med.* 2003;113(1):39-42.

Yen EF, Kane SV, Ladabaum U. Cost-effectiveness of 5-aminosalicylic acid therapy for maintenance of remission in ulcerative colitis. *Am J Gastroenterol.* 2008;103(2):3094-3105.

23

Vaccinations

Sonia Friedman, MD, FACG

Vaccinating patients with IBD is an important part of general care, especially for those patients who are malnourished or taking steroids, immunomodulators, or biologics. Physicians in general underimmunize patients with IBD. Since patients who are immunosuppressed (Table 23-1) have the highest risk of an infection, clinicians must keep patients up to date on their vaccinations. Patients with IBD, especially those on biologics, may not develop high enough antibody titers to be seroprotected, so it is helpful when possible to check postvaccination antibody titers to assess adequate response. In general, patients who are immunosuppressed cannot be given live vaccines (Table 23-2).

I. CONDITIONS TO CONSIDER

- Protein-calorie malnutrition
- Malignant neoplasms of the bone or lymphatic system

Dubinsky M, Friedman S.
Pocket Guide to IBD, Second Edition (pp 169-176).
© 2011 SLACK Incorporated

Table 23-1. Patients Considered Immunocompromised

• Patients treated with glucocorticoids (prednisone >20 mg/day equivalent, or 2 mg/kg/day if less than 10 kg, for 2 weeks or more, and within 3 months of stopping)
• Patients with significant protein-calorie malnutrition
• Patients treated with infliximab/adalimumab/ certolizumab/natalizumab and within 3 months of stopping*
• Patients treated with effective doses of 6-mercaptopurine/ azathioprine and within 3 months of stopping*
• Patients treated with methotrexate and within 3 months of stopping*

*Effect on safety of live vaccines not established.

Table 23-2. Live Vaccines Contraindicated in Patients Receiving Immunosuppressants

Adenovirus types 4 and 7
Anthrax vaccine
Cholera, attenuated, *Vibrio cholerae* strain CVD 103-HgR
Intranasal influenza
Measles-mumps-rubella (MMR)
Polio live oral vaccine (OPV)
Smallpox vaccine
Tuberculosis BCG vaccine
Typhoid live oral vaccine
Varicella
Yellow fever
Zoster*

*Centers for Disease Control and Prevention has recently updated guidelines.

- Acquired immunodeficiency syndrome
- Prednisone therapy
- Azathioprine/6-mercaptopurine (6-MP) therapy
- Methotrexate therapy
- Biologic therapy

II. QUESTIONS TO ASK

Does the patient have antibody titers to the hepatitis B surface antigen, hepatitis A, varicella, and measles-mumps-rubella?

- Patients who are hepatitis B surface antigen (HB$_s$AG) positive need antiviral therapy in conjunction with biologics.
- Blood work for hepatitis A virus (HAV) antibody should be checked and patients vaccinated if they are HAV negative. A booster shot can be given for those already vaccinated but HAV negative.
- Antibodies to measles-mumps-rubella (MMR) should be checked in all patients with IBD. This is especially important in females planning a pregnancy and students in educational institutions.

Is the patient initiating biologic therapy?

- Check for varicella antibodies and vaccinate if needed prior to therapy.

- Check for antibodies to MMR and vaccinate if needed prior to therapy.
- HB$_S$AG should also be drawn. If positive, anti-tumor necrosis factor (anti-TNF) therapy is contraindicated without concomitant antiviral therapy.

Are there any new recommendations for the zoster vaccine?

- The Centers for Disease Control and Prevention (CDC) has recently updated its recommendations for patients on immunosuppressants receiving zoster vaccine. Patients on short courses of prednisone (<14 days, <20 mg/day), those on alternate-day low-dose prednisone, and those on <3 mg/kg of azathioprine, <1.5 mg/kg of 6-MP, or <0.4 mg/kg of methotrexate can now receive the zoster vaccine.

Is the patient a girl or woman aged 9 to 26 years?

- Do not forget about the human papilloma virus vaccine. This vaccine can protect against cervical cancer and should be given to all girls and women between the ages of 9 and 26, especially those on immunomodulators and biologics.

Has the patient had a meningococcal vaccine?

- First-year college students, military recruits, and patients traveling to areas endemic for meningococcemia, such as sub-Saharan Africa, should be vaccinated.

- Patients with asplenia should be vaccinated.

Has the patient had a tetanus booster within the past 10 years?

- Adults should receive a one-time dose of tetanus, diphtheria, and pertussis (Tdap), and then a tetanus and diphtheria (Td) booster every 10 years.

Has the patient had a pneumococcal vaccine polyvalent between the ages of 19 and 26 and then a booster 5 years later?

- All patients with IBD should receive a Pneumovax.

Has the patient had a yearly influenza vaccine?

- The flu shot is the inactivated vaccine and can be safely given.
- Patients on immunosuppressives should *not* receive the intranasal vaccination.

What about the H1N1 vaccine?

- This vaccine is safe in immunocompromised patients. The CDC recommends that the following should be vaccinated:
  - Pregnant women

- ○ People who live with or provide care for children <6 months of age
- ○ Health care and emergency medical services personnel
- ○ People between 6 months and 24 years of age
- ○ People between the ages of 25 and 64 who are at higher risk because of chronic health disorders such as asthma, diabetes, or a weakened immune system

Thus, all patients with IBD and especially those on immunosuppresants and age 24 or younger would qualify.

Will the patient develop antibody titers?

- Patients on anti-TNF therapy may have a slightly decreased immune response and may not be seroprotected with some vaccines. In specific instances, vaccine titers can be checked and booster shots given.

III. TESTS TO ORDER

- HAV antibody and HB$_s$AG
- Varicella titer
- MMR titer

A summary of recommended vaccinations is in Table 23-3.

Table 23-3. Recommended Vaccinations

Tetanus, diphtheria, pertussis (Td/Tdap) (every 10 years)
Human papilloma virus (HPV) (women between the ages of 9 and 26; 3 doses)
Influenza (inactivated vaccine if immunocompromised, yearly)
H1N1 (when available)
Pneumococcal (ages 19 to 26, then in 5 years)
Hepatitis B (3 doses)
Hepatitis A (2 doses)
Meningococcal (for adults with asplenia and those travelling to endemic areas)
Measles-mumps-rubella (MMR) (contraindicated for patients on biologic therapy)
Varicella (2 doses) (if no immunity, give prior to biologic therapy)
Zoster (all adults ages 60 and older; contraindicated for patients on biologic therapy)

SUGGESTED READINGS

Lu Y, Jacobsen D, Bousvaros A. Immunizations in patients with inflammatory bowel disease. *Inflamm Bowel Dis.* 2009;15(9):1417-1423.

Melmed G. Vaccination strategies for patients with inflammatory bowel disease on immunomodulators and biologics. *Inflamm Bowel Dis.* 2009;15(9):1410-1416.

Moscandrew M, Mahadevan U, Kane S. General health maintenance in IBD. *Inflamm Bowel Dis.* 2009;15(9):1399-1409.

National Center for Immunization and Respiratory Diseases, Centers for Disease Control and Prevention. Use of influenza A (H1N1) 2009 monovalent vaccine: recommendations of the advisory committee on immunization practices (ACIP) 2009. *MMWR Recomm Rep.* 2009;58(RR-10):1-8.

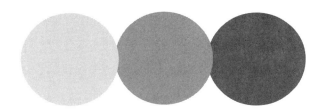

Appendix

Dubinsky M, Friedman S.
Pocket Guide to IBD, Second Edition (pp 177-192).
© 2011 SLACK Incorporated

Medications Used in IBD

Name	Class	FDA IBD Indication	Common Uses	Dosing	Common Adverse Events	Special Considerations
Prednisone, methyl-prednisolone, hydrocortisone	Systemic corticosteroid	None	Moderate to severe UC, CD	1 to 2 mg/kg to a max of 40 to 60 mg orally (or IV) per day	Weight gain, acne, mood changes, puffy face, increased appetite	Not for long-term use; patients doing well on steroids are not in true remission; may affect growth in children
Budesonide (Entocort)	Local-acting corticosteroid	Mild to moderate CD of terminal ileum and colon	Ileocecal CD	9 mg orally for 6 wks, 6 mg for 2 wks, then off	Same as prednisone but occurs less frequently	Safer than prednisone but not for long-term use; used also for collagenous colitis, microscopic colitis

(continued)

Medications Used in IBD (continued)

Name	Class	FDA IBD Indication	Common Uses	Dosing	Common Adverse Events	Special Considerations
Cortifoam, Cortenema, Proctofoam	Topical/rectal steroid	None	Proctitis, active left-sided symptoms	Rectal application 1 to 2 times daily	Weight gain, headache	Some systemic absorption
pH-controlled mesalamine (Asacol)	5-ASA	Mild to moderate UC	Colitis	2.4 to 4.8 g orally (400- or 800-mg tablets)	Headache, diarrhea, abdominal pain	3% to 7% have worsening of colitis
Time-released mesalamine (Pentasa)	5-ASA	Mild to moderate UC	Small and large bowel CD, UC	2 to 4 g orally (250- or 500-mg capsules)	Headache, diarrhea, abdominal pain	3% to 7% have worsening of colitis
MMX mesalamine (Lialda)	5-ASA	Mild to moderate UC	Colitis	2.4 to 4.8 g orally (1.2-g capsules)	Headache, diarrhea, abdominal pain	3% to 7% have worsening of colitis

(continued)

Medications Used in IBD (continued)

Name	Class	FDA IBD Indication	Common Uses	Dosing	Common Adverse Events	Special Considerations
Granular mesalamine (Apriso)	5-ASA	Maintenance of UC	Colitis	1.5 g orally (375-mg capsules)	Headache, diarrhea, abdominal pain	3% to 7% have worsening of colitis
Balsalazide (Colazal)	5-ASA	Mild to moderate UC	Colitis	6.75 g orally (750-mg capsules)	Headache, diarrhea, abdominal pain	3% to 7% have worsening of colitis
Olsalazine (Dipentum)	5-ASA	Maintenance of UC	UC	2 to 3 g orally (500-mg capsules)	Watery diarrhea	None
Sulfasalazine (Azulfidine)	5-ASA	None	Colitis	3 to 6 g orally (500-mg capsules)	Rash, nausea, headache	Folic acid supplementation recommended

(continued)

Medications Used in IBD (continued)

Name	Class	FDA IBD Indication	Common Uses	Dosing	Common Adverse Events	Special Considerations
Mesalamine (Canasa)	Topical 5-ASA	Active ulcerative proctitis	Proctitis	1000 mg rectally once or twice daily (1000-mg suppository)	Bloating, gas	Can be used in combination with oral 5-ASA
Rowasa enema	Topical 5-ASA	Active mild to moderate distal ulcerative colitis, proctosigmoiditis or proctitis	Proctitis, left-sided colitis	4 g per rectum at night (4-g enema)	Bloating, gas, incontinence	Often used in combination with oral 5-ASA
Azathioprine (Azasan, Imuran)	Immuno-modulator	None	More commonly CD but also UC	2 to 2.5 mg/kg body weight orally (50, 75, 100 mg)	Low blood counts, pancreatitis, rash, fevers	Regular blood counts essential for monitoring

(continued)

Medications Used in IBD (continued)

Name	Class	FDA IBD Indication	Common Uses	Dosing	Common Adverse Events	Special Considerations
6-mercapto-purine (Purinethol)	Immuno-modulator	None	Commonly CD but also UC	1 to 1.5 mg/kg body weight orally (50-mg tablets)	Low blood cell counts, pancreatitis, rash, fevers	Regular blood cell counts essential for monitoring
Cyclosporine (Neoral, Sand-immune)	Immuno-modulator	None	Severe UC and CD, fistulizing CD	2 to 4 mg/kg IV then 2x IV dose orally	Hypertension, headache, trem-ors, facial hair growth, low magnesium	Levels need to be monitored to avoid complica-tions; Bactrim for prophylaxis of pneumonia
Methotrexate	Immuno-modulator	None	CD	25-mg injection for 12 wks, then 15-mg maintenance	Mouth ulcers, liver damage, scarring of lungs	Folic acid supplementation recommended; absolutely not used in preg-nancy

(continued)

Medications Used in IBD (continued)

Name	Class	FDA IBD Indication	Common Uses	Dosing	Common Adverse Events	Special Considerations
Tacrolimus (Protopic)	Topical ointment	None	Cutaneous, perineal, perianal CD, pyoderma gangrenosum	Strength 0.03% to 0.1%, apply to affected area once to twice daily	Itching, burning of skin	Minimal absorption, but levels should be monitored initially
Tacrolimus (Prograf)	Immuno-modulator	None	Severe UC and CD, fistulizing CD	0.1 to 0.3 mg/kg/dose orally twice daily	Nausea, heartburn, diarrhea, kidney damage	Levels must be monitored, risks may outweigh potential benefits
Thalidomide	Immuno-modulator	Orphan use for CD	Moderate to severe CD	50 to 250 mg orally daily	Nerve damage, sedation	Never used in pregnancy

(continued)

Medications Used in IBD (continued)

Name	Class	FDA IBD Indication	Common Uses	Dosing	Common Adverse Events	Special Considerations
Ciprofloxacin	Antibiotic	None	Fistulizing and colonic CD	500 to 1000 mg orally daily	Rash, headache, diarrhea	Interacts with nutritional supplements
Metronidazole (Flagyl)	Antibiotic	None	Fistulizing and colonic CD	500 to 1000 mg orally daily	Potential interaction with alcohol, metallic taste, nerve damage	Long-term use often limited by nerve damage, dose reduction may decrease risk
Rifaximin (Xifaxan)	Antibiotic	None	Fistulizing and colonic CD	600 to 1200 mg orally daily	Nausea, diarrhea, abdominal pain	Used for traveler's diarrhea

(continued)

Medications Used in IBD (continued)

Name	Class	FDA IBD Indication	Common Uses	Dosing	Common Adverse Events	Special Considerations
Infliximab (Remicade)	Biologic agent (anti-TNF)	Inflammatory and fistulizing CD, UC	CD, UC, pouchitis, joint and skin problems associated with IBD	5 to 10 mg/kg IV at 0-, 2-, 6-wk induction, then every 8 wks for maintenance	Infusion reactions, delayed hypersensitivity, URI symptoms, other infections	TB test must be performed prior to initiating since increased risk of TB; possible to develop either intolerance or nonresponse over time
Adalimumab (Humira)	Biologic agent (anti-TNF)	Inflammatory CD	Active CD	160 mg, 80-mg qow induction then 40 mg SQ qow	Injection site reactions, infections	PPD must be performed prior to initiating since increased risk of TB; possible to develop either intolerance or nonresponse over time

(continued)

Medications Used in IBD (continued)

Name	Class	FDA IBD Indication	Common Uses	Dosing	Common Adverse Events	Special Considerations
Certolizumab (Cimzia)	Biologic agent (anti-TNF)	Inflammatory CD	Active CD	400 mg SQ wks 2, 4, then every 4 wks	Injection site reactions, infections	PPD must be performed prior to initiating since increased risk of TB; possible to develop either intolerance or nonresponse over time
Natalizumab (Tysabri)	Biologic agent (anti-alpha 4 integrin)	Inflammatory CD	Active CD nonresponsive to other agents	300 mg IV every 4 weeks		Viral brain infection (PML)

ASA indicates aminosalicylate; CD, Crohn's disease; FDA, Food and Drug Administration; IV, intravenous; PML, progressive multifocal leukoencephalopathy; PPD, purified protein derivative; qow, every other week; SQ, subcutaneous; TB, tuberculosis; TNF, tumor necrosis factor; URI, upper respiratory infection.

SUGGESTED READING

Bayless TM, Hanauer SB, eds. *Advanced Therapy of Inflammatory Bowel Disease*. Hamilton, Ontario: BC Decker Incorporated; 2001.

Small Bowel Imaging in Crohn's Disease

Radiographic Study	Sensitivity to Detect Small Bowel Crohn's Disease	Specificity to Detect Small Bowel Crohn's Disease	Uses	Radiographic Exposure	Cons
Small bowel follow through (SBFT)	65% to 72%	94% to 100%	- Detection of small enteric fistulas and sinus tracts - Help assess motility	Yes	- No evaluation of extraenteric complications - Skilled radiologist needed - Incomplete evaluation of pelvic bowel - Incomplete evaluation of post-stricture bowel

(continued)

Small Bowel Imaging in Crohn's Disease (continued)

Radiographic Study	Sensitivity to Detect Small Bowel Crohn's Disease	Specificity to Detect Small Bowel Crohn's Disease	Uses	Radiographic Exposure	Cons
CT enterography (CTE)	82% to 89%	80% to 89%	- Detection of extraluminal complications - Able to distinguish inflammatory from fibrostenotic stenosis	Yes	- Unsafe in pregnancy - Risk of radiation exposure with recurrent use
MR enterography (MRE)	80% to 83%	100%	Comparable to CTE	No	- Motion artifact can hinder study - Patients with prostheses, pacemakers, claustrophobia, etc... are excluded

(continued)

Small Bowel Imaging in Crohn's Disease (continued)

Radiographic Study	Sensitivity to Detect Small Bowel Crohn's Disease	Specificity to Detect Small Bowel Crohn's Disease	Uses	Radiographic Exposure	Cons
Transabdominal ultrasound (TUS)	56% to 94%	67% to 97%	-Noninvasive -Safe for screening for CD complications as well as close follow up post-operative patients	No	-Skilled radiologist needed -Difficulty assessing anorectal disease, proximal small bowel -Inability to detect early disease lesions
Capsule endoscopy (CE)	83%	53%	Higher diagnostic yield for small luminal lesions	No	Lower specificity Need for prior radiographic study to r/o asymptomatic PSBO

(continued)

Small Bowel Imaging in Crohn's Disease (continued)

Radiographic Study	Sensitivity to Detect Small Bowel Crohn's Disease	Specificity to Detect Small Bowel Crohn's Disease	Uses	Radiographic Exposure	Cons
CT Enteroclysis (CTclysis)	77% to 85%	86% to 87%	- Better small bowel distention that CTE - Rest comparable to CTE	Yes	-Invasive as nasojejunal intubation required -Occasional need for conscious sedation -Skilled radiologist needed

Suggested Readings

Chiorean MV, Sandrasegaran K, Saxena R, et al. Correlation of CT enteroclysis with surgical pathology in Crohn's disease. *Am J Gastroenterol.* 2007;102(11): 2541-2550.

Lee S, Kim A, Yang S, et al. Crohn's disease of the small bowel: comparison of CT enterography, MR enterography and small bowel follow through as diagnostic techniques. *Radiology.* 2009;251(3):751-761.

Schmidt S, Felley C, Meuwly JY, et al. CT enteroclysis: technique and clinical applications. *Eur Radiol.* 2006;16(3):648-660.

Solem CA, Loftus EV Jr, Fletcher JG, et al. Small bowel imaging in Crohn's disease: a prospective, blinded, 4-way comparison trial. *Gastrointest Endosc.* 2008;68(2): 255-266.

Financial Disclosures

Dr. Maria T. Abreu is a consultant for Abbott, AMGEN, Elan, Eisai, Opsona, Prometheus, Salix Pharmaceuticals Laboratories, Millenium/Takeda, and UCB.

Dr. David G. Binion received honoraria and grant support and is a consultant for UCB.

Dr. Russel D. Cohen is a consultant for Proctor & Gamble Pharmaceuticals, Salix Pharmaceuticals, Shire, and Warner-Chilcott. He gives lectures for MSD Brazil, Salix Pharmaceuticals, and Shire.

Dr. Judy F. Collins received grant support from Centocor Ortho Biotech, and UCB. She is a consultant for UCB and is part of the speaker's bureau for Salix Pharmaceuticals.

Dr. Marla Dubinsky has received research support from Centocor Ortho Biotech and UCB. She is a consultant for Prometheus, Abbott, UCB, and Shire.

Dr. Sandra M. El-Hachem has no financial or proprietary interest in the materials presented herein.

Dr. Erin Feldman has no financial or proprietary interest in the materials presented herein.

Dr. Sonia Friedman has no financial or proprietary interest in the materials presented herein.

Dr. Matthew J. Hamilton has no financial or proprietary interest in the materials presented herein.

Dr. Debra J. Helper has no financial or proprietary interest in the materials presented herein.

Dr. Sarah N. Horst has no financial or proprietary interest in the materials presented herein.

Dr. Kim L. Isaacs receives grant support from Millenium/Takeda, Centocor Ortho Biotech, UCB, Elan, and Abbott. She is on a data safety monitoring board for Centocor Ortho Biotech.

Dr. Sunanda V. Kane is a consultant for Abbott, Elan, Millenium/Takeda, Shire, and Warner-Chilcott. She has received research support from Elan and Shire.

Dr. Joshua Korzenik has received research support from Warner-Chilcott and Proctor & Gamble.

Dr. Edward V. Loftus is a consultant for Abbott, UCB, and Bristol-Myers Squibb. He has received research support from Abbott, UCB, Amgen, Centocor Ortho Biotech Ortho Biotech, Millenium/Takeda, and Shire.

Dr. Uma Mahadevan is a consultant for Biogen, Gilead, Centocor Ortho Biotech, Abbott, UCB, and Elan.

Dr. Nimisha K. Parekh has no financial or proprietary interest in the materials presented herein.

Dr. Kris Radcliff has no financial or proprietary interest in the materials presented herein.

Dr. David T. Rubin received grant support from Proctor & Gamble and Salix Pharmaceuticals. He is a consultant for Axcan, Proctor & Gamble, Shire, and Salix Pharmaceuticals.

Dr. Ellen J. Scherl has received research or grant support from Abbott, Centocor Ortho Biotech, Cerimon, Elan, Prometheus, Salix Pharmaceuticals, UCB, Genotech, and Millenium/Takeda. She is a consultant or on the advisory board/speaker's bureau for Abbott, AstraZeneca, Axcan, Berlex, Centocor Ortho Biotech, Cerimon, Crohn's & Colitis Foundation of America, PDL, Proctor & Gamble, Prometheus Laboratories, Questcor Pharmaceuticals, Salix Pharmaceuticals, Shire, Sigma Tau Pharmaceuticals, Inc, Solvay, TAP Pharmaceuticals, and UCB. She has received an honorarium from Abbott, AstraZeneca, Axcan, Centocor Ortho Biotech, Cerimon, Proctor & Gamble, PDL, Prometheus Laboratories, Salix Pharmaceuticals, Shire, Sigma Tau Pharmaceuticals, Inc, Solvay, TAP Pharmaceuticals, and UCB. She has also received other financial or material support from Centocor Ortho Biotech, Salix Pharmaceuticals, Abbott, Prometheus, Crohn's & Colitis Foundation of America, PDL, and UCB.

Dr. David A. Schwartz is a consultant for P&G, Abbott, Centocor Ortho Biotech, Salix Pharmaceuticals, UCB, Prometheus, Cellerix, Shire, Axcan. He has received grant support from P&G, Abbott, and UCB.

Dr. Bo Shen received a research grant from Ocera, an education grant from UCB, and is a consultant for Prometheus.

Index